Milica Vladova

BUILD YOUR

IMMUNE SYSTEM

FAST:

Proven Immune Boosters, Healthy Anti-cancer Recipes, Homeopathic Remedies, Probiotic Yogurt Recipes, Herbal Tea, and more

Milica Vladova
"Build Your Immune System Fast: Proven Immune Boosters, Healthy Anti-cancer Recipes, Homeopathic Remedies, Probiotic Yogurt Recipes, Herbal Tea, and more"

ISBN-13: 978-1981150267

ISBN-10: 1981150269

This book is not intended as a substitute for the medical advice of physicians. The reader should regularly consult a physician in matters relating to his/her health and particularly with respect to any symptoms that may require diagnosis or medical attention. The information I share in this book is based on my personal experience, conclusions, observations and studies. I am not a medical professional, nor a health expert. Before implementing any of the information shared in this book, consult with your physician or nutritionist! No information in this book should be used to diagnose, treat, prevent or cure any disease or condition.By reading this book, you acknowledge that you are responsible for your own health decisions. Do not take anything from this book and try it without proper research and medical supervision. The author does not assume any responsibility for any injuries or accidents.

FREE EBOOKS

Strengthen your immunity, detox, energize, heal, and stimulate your metabolism with these magical potent healthy recipes!

Get your FREE copy of
"***10 Powerful Immune Boosting Recipes***"
"12 Healthy Dessert Recipes"
"15 Delicious & Healthy Smoothies"
"The Complete Ayurveda Detox"

Go to ***www.MindBodyAndSpiritWellbeing.com*** and claim your book!

Or simply scan the QR code below:

Dedicated to my mother.

Thank you for your support, care, and love!

Thank you for always believing in me!

Contents

Basic Immune Boosting Principles

"A good laugh and a long sleep are the best cures in the doctor's book."

~Irish Proverb

Let's cover the basics here and get them out of the way. After all, we need to create the proper basis for all other specific immune boosting techniques and recipes covered later in the book. It may turn out that all our defense system needed was more sleep or some sunlight. Here is what you can do to build a stronger natural immunity from today:

- **Do not take any antibiotics** (or any other type of medications) **if not absolutely necessary.** Do not self-medicate with these strong medications and always consult with your physician beforehand. They will guide you in the right direction and make a judgment whether the antibiotics are applicable for your case or not. Later in the book you will find out how serious this matter is, and why these meds should not be underestimated.
- **Try to keep a healthy diet as much as you can.** Avoid highly processed foods, and drinks, full of chemicals.
- **Wear comfortable clothes that do not press against your body** – they hamper the blood and lymph flow and can cause lots of serious damage to our systems.

- **Take frequent walks outside among a clean environment**, if possible. The direct sunlight stimulates the production of vitamin D, essential for our immunity. This is one of the reasons why we get ill more often during the winter. Remember to apply non-toxic sunscreen.
- **Stay active** – engage in some sort of moderate physical activity (fast walking, jogging, dancing, yoga, qi gong, etc.). It stimulates the blood and lymph flow, and creates a positive type of stress that naturally pushes our bodies to become more adaptable.
- **Take contrasting showers** – the logic behind this is the same – we create a small temperature shock that makes the body stronger and more versatile. Just remember to start slowly – for just a couple of minutes a day during your daily shower. Slowly adjust the temperature of the water so the body won't be shocked too much. Always end the contrasting showers with cold water.
- **Take vitamins, minerals and enzymes** – it is best if they come straight from the food - from lots of fresh fruits and veggies. But if you feel you do not take enough of the daily recommendations, some additional organic supplements will do. It is always a good idea to take some blood tests and see how your parameters are doing and to check if there is anything missing.
- **Have enough sleep** – the duration depends on the individual, but the general rule is that if you need any stimulants (like coffee or energy drinks) in the morning, you do not sleep enough. In book one you will get some specific strategies for overcoming the caffeine addiction and learn some ideas for healthy coffee

substitutes. Also, avoid reading, working on your laptop or watching TV in the bed – we need to create a specific association with the bed, which is sleep and nothing else.

- **Avoid using harsh chemicals on your body and your environment.** In "Toxin-free Homemade Easy Beauty Recipes" you will get tons of ideas for your natural healthy body care, plus some recipes for your toxin-free sunscreen.
- **Stay positive as much as possible**. It is scientifically proven that people with a positive outlook are healthier. Smiling, laughing, hugging, kissing, and even having sex, stimulate the production of "happy" hormones, lower the stress levels and boost the immunity.

Probiotics and immunity

"He who takes medicine and neglects to diet wastes the skill of his doctors."

~Chinese Proverb

It is a well-known fact that our intestines play an important role in our immunity. As trite as this can sound, most diseases indeed come from the intestines (as Hippocrates would say). And one of the main reasons is our gut flora. Our digestive system is inhabited with more than 100 trillion (yes, trillion!) bacteria – beneficial and malevolent. If both types are living in a natural balance – about 85% beneficial and 15% non-beneficial – our system and our immunity are doing fine. The good colon bacteria can handle and suppress the growth of the malevolent microorganisms that cause diseases and discomforts. They also act as immune regulators – they prepare the walls of the intestines to absorb the nutrients and stimulate the production of essential vitamins like A, B, and K. These little, but very important, allies even produce their own natural antibiotics that kill the bad flora and prevent it from overgrowing.

Unfortunately, our current lifestyle is not so good to this loyal guarding army (too much stress, frequent usage of antibiotics, radiation, unhealthy diet, etc.) tends to harm the beneficial colon flora and stimulate the growth the malevolent types. This leads to a condition called dysbacteriosis (also dysbiosis), which manifests as gastrointestinal issues (constipation, diarrhea, irritable bowel syndrome, flatulence), low immunity and frequent colds and the flu, not to mention the development of serious illnesses on the long run. A lot of medical scientists support the thesis that most diseases (including cancer) are the result of intestinal dysbiosis.

The latest researches show that our natural defense system counteracts the pathogens using a group of proteins called interferons. Interferons suppress the development of the disease by destroying the infected cells and preventing from further spreading of the viruses in our bodies. That is how our natural processes of self-defense and self-recovery are boosted and sped up. So, how do we make sure we have (and produce) enough interferons? The answer is simple – by taking care of our intestinal microflora. The beneficial colon bacteria boost and support the natural development of interferons.

Another research (concentrated on the diet of centenarians) shows one thing in common – they all have natural high levels of beneficial gut flora. As we get old leading a stressful and unhealthy lifestyle, we tend to harm our good bacteria and the results quickly become visible – fatigue, low immunity, and frequent illnesses. So, the first steps for a healthier and a more vibrant long life is making positive lifestyle changes and ensuring our gut flora is balanced and in a good condition. How can we do this? In this chapter I will share with you lots of options and ideas for replenishing your good intestinal flora and boosting your natural immunity.

What kills my beneficial colon bacteria?

"Health is a relationship between you and your body"
~Terri Guillemets

When talking about immunity, longevity, and health, one of the first things we need to look at is our gastrointestinal tract. As I said before – healthy gut, healthy you! So, our first task will be to take care of our intestinal microflora, to replenish it and to make sure we keep it healthy and balanced. Now let's take a look at what are the most common culprits for damaged colon bacteria (dysbiosis). Our goal will be to start making changes and establish habits that will prevent from harming these healthy guests on the long run.

1. ***Antibiotics***

   This is the number 1 reason why we have low immunity and relapsing (and even chronic) illnesses, especially viral infections. The antibiotic treatments can be vital for our survival, but nowadays they have been over-abused and used for minor health cases. The result is more resilient pathogenic bacteria (becoming superbacteria), low immunity, and chronic gastrointestinal issues.

   An excellent example is the ultimate female menace – the vaginal infection with Candida. When the discomforts begin, you go to your gynecologist and they prescribe you an antibiotic. The symptoms subside, but in a while the problems continue – either another Candida infection or other health issues from the hampered immunity – colds, the flu, sore throat, tonsillitis, flatulence, constipation, etc. Sadly, these conditions are frequently treated with antibiotics (again!) and the cycle continues until one day the antibiotic treatment just stops working. And the moral of the story is to use antibiotics responsibly and as a last resort. I highly recommend you find a holistic physician or a GP who supports natural health practices. They will be able to guide you in the right direction with fewer "hard" pharmaceuticals and with a more natural gentle approach.

Keep in mind that the antibiotics are not the only pharmaceuticals that suppress and destroy the beneficial colon bacteria. Sulfonamides, hormone supplements, and harsh laxatives should also be added to the list. ***A replenishing gut flora course should always be administered after such treatments.***

2. ***Too much stress***

We are all too stressed these days and this is harming our health and lowers our immunity. There are mainly two types of stress – positive and negative. The positive stress is everything that "shocks" our bodies and makes them adjust and evolve. Excellent examples are working out and intermittent fasting. But when the stressful circumstances evoke strong negative emotions (like fear or anger) for a long period of time, the stress becomes very unhealthy. Our bodies work constantly in a fight-or-flight mode producing lots of stress hormones (cortisol, adrenaline). Since our survival is one of the top high priority tasks for our brain, it becomes occupied with hormone secretion and preparing for defense (or attack). The production of lymphocytes (the cells which are responsible for our immunity) goes in the background. As a result, constant stress makes us more vulnerable and susceptible to various diseases, especially stomach ulcers, gastritis, colitis, IBS, etc.

3. ***Unhealthy diet***

By feeding ourselves, we also feed those little beneficial microorganisms as well. This means that if our diet is poor, we slowly destroy them and suppress their natural growth. It is a perfect symbiosis in which by taking care of ourselves, we take care of our gut flora allies, too. What does a unhealthy diet mean? It means not taking enough natural whole foods, lack of essential nutrients, vitamins, minerals, enzymes; taking too much artificial additives, preservatives, colorings, strong toxins like alcohol and tobacco, etc. So, the first steps into getting back our natural immunity is to look at our plate and put some healthy foods in it! If you have trouble figuring out how to make that change more tolerable and achievable, go to book 1of this series ("Healthy Body Cleanse") and get some ideas.

4. ***Parasites***

Humanity has made a huge progress with regards to personal hygiene and prevention. Unfortunately, we still have not managed to get rid of parasites completely. These small harmful guests are robbing us from essential nutrients and damaging our immunity for a long time without us suspecting anything at all! That is why a regular (for example annually) parasite detox is an important part of keeping our bodies healthy, and our beneficial colon bacteria – alive and kicking! Although parasite cleansing sounds gross and difficult, it actually can be very easy and simple. Hop in to book 2 ("Complete Body Cleansing") and find some interesting and effective ways to keep these unwelcomed guests away from your body temple!

5. ***Sleep deprivation***

It is not a secret that most people are chronically deprived of enough sleep. From working long hours to being glued to the TV late in the evening, we all have or have had some issues with getting enough sleep. We just gulp another sip of strong black coffee and keep going. This fragrant dark liquid pumps the heart, alerts us for a while, but ultimately disrupts our circadian rhythm and natural sleep patterns. The result is – we feel lethargic and groggy during the day and wide awake in the evening. We keep extending our go-to-bed time, wake up tired and pour the regular cup of morning coffee, and the vicious cycle continues... No wonder all sleep deprivation related diseases are increasing at a racing pace these days. And the symptoms begin with a lowered immunity, exhaustion, more and more frequents colds, leading to more serious ailments. No matter how simple or even ridiculous it sounds, make sure you make sleep a priority. Another good life vest will be to start taking some afternoon naps to catch enough zzz's.

6. ***Not enough sun light***

This is not directly connected to the intestinal flora, but it is essential for our immunity. When we expose to natural sun light, our bodies produce the active vitamin D - indispensable for the proper Calcium absorption. The ultraviolet rays also directly kill the malevolent microorganisms and stimulate the production of white "killer" cells (lymphocytes). That is why the cold seasons are such a challenge for our immunity – on one hand, the low temperatures shock the body and cause stress, and on the other – the lack of sun naturally decreases our defense system's abilities. Another side of the problem is that now most people lead very sedentary lives, working in offices under artificial lights. Needless to say, this is not enough exposure to the Sun to activate the immune system. That is why try to spend enough time outside whenever you can. ***Important: direct exposure to the Sun should be done responsibly and with a proper sunscreen, especially between 11:00 AM and 16:00 PM. Pay extra attention to the UV protection during the summer and when snowing.***

7. ***Low personal hygiene***

The truth is that the microorganisms are all around us. Having an absolutely clean environment is impossible and not even healthy. But we need to make sure we keep our bodies frequently disinfected, especially during the cold seasons. If we load the immunity with too many toxins, it may not be able to tackle all of its tasks. So, it is best if we do our part and keep top notch hygiene. Here is an interesting recipe with essential oils, to keep malevolent microorganisms away! It is called "*The Four Thieves' Oil*". The legend goes back to the Middle Ages when the plague became epidemic. The four thieves decided to rob the homes of the people who died from the Black Death. No one would even come close to their homes out of fear of contamination. But these four dodgers were former spice merchants and knew the wonderful healing and disinfecting properties of essential oils. So, they created a blend that will keep them from catching the plague. Here is the recipe itself:

The Four Thieves' Oil

Ingredients:
40 drops **cloves essential oil**
35 drops **lemon essential oil**
20 drops **cinnamon essential oil**
15 drops **eucalyptus essential oil**
10 drops **rosemary essential oil**
Carrier oil of choice – from almonds, avocados, coconuts, jojoba, etc.

Directions:

Mix all essential oils in a dark glass bottle. If you have one with a droplet, even better. Dilute 6-12 drops of the blend in 2 Tbsps. carrier oil, stir, and the mixture is ready for rubbing on the hands or body.

You can even mix some of the blend with some water in a spray bottle and make your own universal disinfecting and refreshing spray. The essential oils must be about 1% of the water quantity.

8. Other

These were the main seven reasons why our gut flora might be hampered. But beyond them, there are some other culprits that should be mentioned and taken into account. For example, surgeries (especially those connected to the intestines), too much physical strain (working out too hard without giving time for the body to recover), intestinal infections (such as dysentery), issues with the digestive tract (stomach, pancreas, etc.), thyroid health issues, poor environment (contaminated water, air, radiation), chemotherapy, and so on.

Replenishing the gut flora naturally

"A man too busy to take care of his health is like a mechanic too busy to take care of his tools."
~Spanish Proverb

If you suspect your gut flora is not doing well, you have undergone some of the treatments mentioned above, or you just need to regularly boost your natural immunity, read on! This section is dedicated to finding and applying simple techniques and recipes that will help us recover our beneficial gut bacteria and restore our health and vitality! Here are some telltale signs your gut flora might need some boosting:

- *Frequent bloating and flatulence;*
- *Chronic constipation and/or diarrhea;*
- *Stomach reflux and burping;*
- *Nausea and vomiting;*
- *High stomach acidity;*
- *Bad breath;*
- *Overall gastrointestinal discomfort and pains;*
- *Chronic fatigue and lost appetite;*
- *Food allergies, etc.*

In case you have some or all of these symptoms, consult with your physician and avoid self-medicating and self-diagnosing!

Now let's get back to replenishing the gut flora. The process is simple but it needs some of your patience and persistence! Here is what you can do, but remember that

Rome was not built in a day! This process needs at least one month to have some profound effect!

1. ***First things first***

    If you are recovering from an antibiotic treatment or any other harsh invasive operation, you need to counteract the damage to the gut flora. And homeopathy has the best tool for this purpose! Even if you are not keen on homeopathy, you still can give it a try – it is considered safe and cannot be overdosed. ***However, if you have high blood sugar level, or any other disease, consult with your physician and homeopathic specialist beforehand!***

    The remedy we will be using is *Thuya (Thuya Occidentalis)* - this is the ultimate homeopathic remedy for recovering from antibiotics, corticosteroids, and cytostatics. It can also prevent from negative side effects from vaccines. Take ***5 granules Thuya 9CH a day 3 days in the week*** – Tuesday, Thursday, and Saturday for at least a month.

    Another first-aid homeopathic remedy for counteracting the negative effect from antibiotics and supporting the beneficial colon bacteria growth is *Monilia albicans*. This is a homeopathic product, which is suitable for fighting and preventing from fungal infections as well. Like the Thuya, ***take 5 granules Monilia albicans 15CH a day three days of the week*** for at least a month. The days must be different. If you take Thuya on Tuesday, Thursday and Saturday, take Monilia on Monday, Wednesday and Friday.

2. *Adding prebiotics*

The prebiotics are very important for our natural gut flora. These are types of carbohydrates that stimulate the growth and health of these precious beneficial colon bacteria. In other words, we feed the gut flora by ingesting the foods they like. Most of these substances are not digestible for us (like cellulose), but they certainly have an essential role in our strong immunity. Start including more asparagus, bananas, onions, garlic, fresh cabbage, white beans, bran (oat, rice, and wheat bran), artichoke, apples, carrots, turnip, beetroot, leek, etc. in your diet.

3. *Adding probiotics*

We can stimulate the growth of the colon bacteria, but if the process is not fast and powerful enough, we can start adding the probiotics themselves. This way we work in both directions – replenishing the gut flora and creating a welcoming environment for their existence. If you are not familiar with probiotics, these are the good bacteria themselves. Fortunately, they can be found in lots of foods and food supplements. For example, kefir, miso, sauerkraut, Bulgarian yogurt (the only one containing the Lactobacillus Bulgaricus probiotic), gouda, pickles, sourdough bread, etc. Of course, you can buy high quality probiotic supplements that can assist you with the right dosages of the bacteria. Pay special attention to the colostrum supplements, they are extremely beneficial for our immunity and gastrointestinal tract.

Natural prebiotics

"An apple a day keeps the doctor away"

~Proverb

We have discussed what prebiotics are and why they are so important for our immunity. Let's just sum it up. The prebiotics are the food for the probiotics. These are nutrients in our meals that serve as growth stimulators for the beneficial colon bacteria. In return, the gut flora boosts our immunity and stimulates our healthy digestion. The prebiotic substances are mainly fiber which we cannot digest (unlike ruminants). But this fiber plays an essential role in physically cleaning up any food debris in the colon and as food for the good colon bacteria. Not any fiber is a prebiotic. To be classified as such, the fiber should not be broken down by our digestion, to ferment in the guts, and selectively stimulate the growth of the beneficial gut flora. Since the medical science discovered this wonderful health effect of these nutrients, it started researching which substances have this immune building effect. For now the list consists of inulin, oligofructose, fructo-oligosaccharides, galacto-oligosaccharides, and other oligosaccharides. The best known and researched are inulin and the oligofructose. They serve as food for different beneficial bacterial colonies in different segments of the guts. That is why it is best for us to take and combine various types of prebiotics.

What other benefits hold the prebiotics?

The prebiotic substances are not just immune boosters. They have been proven to affect our health in various ways. For example, studies show that increased consumption of these foods (mainly in fruits and veggies), improve the absorption of essential minerals like Calcium and Magnesium. Also, it beneficially affects people with insulin resistance and high cholesterol levels. And that's not all! Thanks to the prebiotics, the production of specific fatty acids is stimulated in the guts. These fatty acids regulate the blood sugar level and act as adaptogens (improve our stress management). Another excellent effect from taking prebiotics regularly is their gentle support of natural weight-loss. It has been discovered that prebiotics have the power to suppress the appetite. That is why in book 1 of The Healthy Detox and Strong Immunity Series, I mentioned how important it is to take enough fiber and substitute white flour with healthier alternatives. The wholegrain products contain natural prebiotics, they are much healthier, they are digested slowly, do not raise the blood sugar level rapidly, and do not ruin your slender physique. And as it turns out – they boost your immunity as well.

Where to find more prebiotics?

Naturally, prebiotics can be found in fruits and veggies with lots of fiber. The recommended daily amount is 4-16 grams prebiotics. Here is a list of foods that can supply lots of these healthy nutrients in copious amounts. To supply 6 grams of prebiotics, you need to take:

- 10 grams (0.35 o.z.) **chicory roots**
- 20 grams (0.70 o.z.) **topinambur**
- 30 grams (1.06 o.z.) **sorrel**
- 35 grams (1.23 o.z.) **garlic**
- 40 grams (1.40.o.z.) **leek**
- 70 grams (2.46 o.z.) **onion (raw)**
- 120 grams (4.20 o.z.) **onions (cooked)**
- 500 grams (17.60 o.z.) **bananas**

If you do not like these options, you can munch on radish, artichoke, asparagus, avocados, oat meal, barley, wheat germ, etc.

It is best to take these foods raw, because the prebiotic substances break down during heat treatment (especially inulin). Another excellent option is to prepare some homemade pickles and combine the power of prebiotics and probiotics. You can find such potent recipe in the free ebook “10 Powerful Immune Boosting Recipes”.

Here is another prebiotic recipe you can try for boosting your natural defense system in the cold season:

Winter Spicy Salad

Ingredients (for 2 portions):
2 big **carrots**
1/2 bulb **white radish**
4-5 small bulbs **topinambur**
3-4 cm. (1.2-1.6 inch.) **horseradish root**
1 apple
2 Tbsps. **sour cream**
Some **Himalayan salt**

Directions:

Grate the carrots, radish, topinambur, and the apple using the large holes of the grater. For the horseradish, on the other hand, use the fine grater. Mix the ingredients in a bowl, add the sour cream and the salt and mix well.

Enjoy!

Natural probiotics

"True healthcare reform starts in your kitchen, not in Washington"

~Anonymous

As we have discussed in the previous chapter, we need to supply our digestive system with fresh beneficial colon bacteria regularly. Because no matter how healthy we try to live, there are always some factors that disrupt the gut flora's balance. And it is our responsibility to keep it in a good shape. The most convenient way, of course, is to buy ready-made probiotic supplements from the pharmacy. And in severe cases of dysbiosis, this may be a step that cannot be skipped. We can stimulate the growth of the bacteria and keep them balanced with natural tools, but the path will be much quicker with these small capsules full of the good gut flora. Pay extra attention to the colostrum&probiotic combined supplements. They can be invaluable for boosting the immunity after long antibiotic treatments, radiation, chemotherapy, etc. Consult with your physician to point you at the right direction and recommend you a high quality probiotic remedy.

Colostrum

Let's talk a little bit more about the colostrum and why it is extremely important to breastfeed and build our kids' immunity right from the start.

The colostrum is the first breast milk fluid that comes out of the mammary glands. It is produced mainly in the first 3-4 days after childbirth and it becomes our first food. It is extremely important and indispensable for the young organism – colostrum contains around 37 natural immune substances and 8 growth stimulators!

Colostrum was widely used for preventive and healing purposes back in the day. Cow colostrum is especially praised and used even today in India. A while ago, many medical researches were commenced to unveil the magical powers of this immune boosting substance. But as the era of antibiotics began, the main focus shifted elsewhere. Now, as we begin to see the detrimental long-term effect of antibiotics, we must go back and seek the benefits of probiotics and prebiotics. And colostrum is one of the most powerful of them all.

How does colostrum affect our bodies?

The beneficial effects of mother's first breast milk are numerous. As we discovered earlier, its goal is to strengthen the baby's body, build its natural defense mechanisms, promote its rapid growth, and help it survive. Here is a short summary of colostrum's benefits on humans:

- *It protects the fragile newborn from its first days of life.*
- *Promotes muscle growth.*
- *Regulates the body mass.*
- *Protects the body from bacteria, fungi, viruses, and infections.*
- *Promotes the normal growth and development of the body.*
- *Strengthens the bones and their density.*
- *Boosts the stamina and physical strength.*

- *Increases the endurance and performance.*
- *Speeds the self-healing recovery processes.*
- *Fights anxiety and prevents from mood swings.*
- *Slows down the aging process and rejuvenates the body.*
- *Has a natural lifting and anti-wrinkle effect.*
- *Promotes longevity.*
- *Lowers and balances the blood sugar level.*
- *Soothes various types of allergies.*
- *Builds a strong immunity, and many more.*

How does this simple pale white liquid can do all these essential things?

The answer is within its contents. Colostrum is packed with compounds and natural substances that boost our organism from day 1. For example:

- **Vitamins** – A, B1, B2, B5, B6, B9, B12, C, E, Beta-carotene, retinoic acid, riboflavin, etc.
- **Minerals** – Sodium, Chrome, Zinc, Magnesium, Calcium, Phosphorus, Potassium, etc.
- **Special chemical factors** – **immunoglobulin** (this factor neutralizes the viruses and toxins in the gastrointestinal and respiratory tracts), **cytokines** (boost the immune system for the long term), lactoferrin (this is a special milk protein that protects us from viruses and malevolent microorganisms), **interleukin 10** (a special compound that slows down and counteracts inflammations), **polypeptide** (a prolin rich hormone which stimulates the thymus gland), **oligo-polysaccharides and glycoconjugates** (simple sugars that fight the pathogenic bacteria

and keep them from entering the stomach), **epithelial tissue growth factor** (a.k.a. EGF - stimulates the recovery of the tissues and stomach ulcers), **Insulin-like growth factor** (a.k.a. EGF-1 – essential for the growth of the muscle and bone tissue), **transforming growth factors** (a.k.a. TGF A & B – stimulates the recovery of all kinds of wounds and harmed tissues), **growth hormone** (important for the normal development of the human body to its full genetic potential), and more.

Now you see why colostrum is so important, and why breastfeeding our kids from day 1 is critical for their development as human beings. But babies are not the only ones who can benefit from this powerful probiotic natural remedy! As we grow older, our system needs regular boosting and support. And colostrum (combined with a healthy diet) can have a tremendous immune strengthening, anti-aging, and rejuvenating effects! You can soothe the inflammation from rheumatoid arthritis, prevent and recover from osteoporosis, fight obesity and high blood sugar with this simple food additive. It even can be used as a powerful assistant in counteracting serious health cases like transplant surgeries, cancer, and AIDS. Consult with your physician beforehand.

Kefir

Kefir is a healthy natural dairy drink full of probiotics and beneficial nutrients. It originates from the Caucasus mountain region and it is well known and used by the Tibetan and Mongolian tribes. Now this precious healthy product has gained a lot of popularity and spread all around the world.

What is kefir?

Kefir and its production look very similar to the normal yogurt – it is made from milk (goat, cow, sheep) and milk yeast grains (probiotic bacteria that coagulate the milk proteins). When you mix the main two components, leave them to ferment at room temperature, and stir/shake them occasionally, you will get a nice sour, slightly carbonated and alcoholic probiotic drink. Do not worry, though, the alcoholic amount is very low – not more than 1%. Be aware that the homemade kefir made by the traditional recipes will be very different from the store bought products.

Why kefir is so beneficial?

If you prepare your kefir with natural bio milk and high quality yeast, you will get a dairy product packed with nutrients, vitamins, minerals, and probiotics that will boost your organism. After all, remember that kefir is used by the people living in very harsh regions and this dairy drink supports their bodies and build their immunity. The typical kefir contains:

- *More than 10 types of beneficial microorganisms and bacteria;*
- *Tryptophan amino acid;*
- *Milk protein (casein) and polysaccharides;*
- *Biotin (helps with the absorption of the group B vitamins);*
- *Vitamins A, B1, B2, B6, D, K2, folic acid;*
- *Minerals such as Calcium, Iron, and Iodine.*

Kefir is a balanced and healthy food you can safely include in your diet. It will have many benefits for your body and mind. It is suitable for people of all ages who want to boost their immunity and supply their organisms with lots of essential substances. Kefir is proven to have various beneficial effects:

- *It is easily digested and* ***gently cleans the bowels;***
- ***Soothes the nervous system*** *and helps people relieve anxiety, depression, insomnia, hyperactivity, etc.*
- ***Supports the digestive system*** *– regulates the bowel movement, soothes bloating and flatulence, and other stomach issues;*
- ***Supplies lots of digestible Calcium****, boosts the bone development in children and prevents from osteoporosis in adults;*
- *The probiotics in kefir* ***replenish the beneficial colon bacteria*** *and fight various bacterial infections (like the widespread and stubborn Candida);*
- ***Regulates the blood pressure;***
- ***Supports the heart*** *and the overall cardiovascular system;*
- ***Regulates the digestion;***
- ***Soothes IBS and colitis;***
- ***Balances the stomach acidity*** *(excellent for people with reflux), and more…*

Important: if your gut flora is highly imbalanced, you can experience some negative side effects from the homemade quality kefir. This is the reaction of the body adapting to the new flora. It may cause some

flatulence or even diarrhea. In this case, start with small amounts in the evening until the body gets used to the beneficial probiotics. In case you have any health issues (especially regarding the kidneys or the liver), consult with your physician. Once the digestion adjusts to the micro flora, the side effects will subside.

How to prepare your own kefir at home?

You can buy kefir in most health stores, but it is always best to make it on your own. That is how you have full control of the ingredients and make sure everything is high quality. Let's begin!

First you need to find kefir grains. You can buy them or ask a friend to give you some. Do not worry - after the fermentation process, the grains can double their size. So, every fan of kefir will have plenty to share.

The next ingredient is, of course, milk. Make sure it is as high quality as possible – from grass fed animals, preferably not treated with hormones and antibiotics.

Also you will need a large glass jar, plastic strainer or cheesecloth, and a wooden spoon. ***Do not use any metal utensils!***

Mix the kefir grains and the milk in the jar at approximate 1:10 ratio. Seal the jar and place it in a warm room or in a special yogurt maker to keep the temperature steady and high enough. In about 24-48 hours the kefir drink should be ready. You will know when the product is ready by these signs: *when you open the jar, you can hear a slight pop, like opening a soda; the milk has become thicker (jelly-like), but it still has liquid consistency; it has a slightly carbonated taste, like a dairy soda.*

After the dairy product is ready, strain it and save the remaining kefir grains for your next use.

It is important to store the grains carefully. The best way is to mix them with some milk in a glass jar (do not fill the jar to the top) and store it in the fridge. In 5-6 days change the milk. If you cannot maintain them in this way, you can dry the grains and place them in dry milk. When you decide to make kefir again, wash the grains with pure water and place them in some milk again. It will quickly reactive the probiotics.

If you do not like milk or if you are lactose intolerant, you can try this next recipe and still benefit from the wonderful kefir.

Lactose-free Coconut Kefir

Ingredients:
7 cups **coconut water**
5 Tbsps. **kefir grains**

Directions:

Put the coconut water in a glass jar and add the kefir grains. Let the mixture sit at room temperature for about 2 days. When the grains ferment (they will pop on top of the water and float), the kefir is ready.

Strain the mixture and it is ready for consumption. Remember to soak the kefir grains in some milk to keep them alive or dry them, if you do not intent to use them any time soon.

This recipe is excellent for lactose intolerant people who want to avoid consuming any dairy products. It combines the powers of two extremely beneficial products – coconut water and kefir. Coconut water is one of the best liquids for the human body. It is an electrolyte drink, which supplies us with essential minerals and nutrients – vitamins A, B6, C, E, K; Potassium, Magnesium, Calcium, Sodium, beta-carotene, riboflavin, niacin, pantothenic acid, folic acid, and more. It nourishes our cells, hydrates us and builds our natural immunity. Coconut water is very similar to the human's blood plasma, it even can be used as an emergency substitute!

Bulgarian yogurt

Bulgarian yogurt is not like the other types you can find on the market. The fermentation of the milk is caused by a special type of bacterium that cannot be found anywhere except Bulgarian air. That is why it is called Lactobacillus Bulgaricus. It gives the Bulgarian yogurt its distinct taste, flavor and beneficial properties. The other important ingredient is Streptococcus thermophiles. Combined, these probiotics cause the coagulation of the lactose and turn it into our famous sour milk (yogurt).

Traditional Bulgarian yogurt, made from organic pure milk, is one of the best dietary additions to your healthy meals. It has numerous benefits and perks. It contains:

- *Easily digestible* ***dairy protein*** *(casein);*
- ***Special probiotics*** *(Lactobacillus Bulgaricus), which are the only type in the world (known to man) that have*

only positive effects on us and do not harm the human body in any way;

- *Wide variety of* ***vitamins*** *- A, B, C, D, E, F;*
- *Essential minerals and* ***microelements*** *– Potassium, Sodium, Calcium, Iodine, Iron, Cobalt, Zinc, Nickel, etc.*
- ***Low amounts of lactose.*** *If the yogurt is produced with organic pure goat milk, the amount of lactose is even lower. This makes it a perfect healthy meal for people with lactose intolerance and respiratory issues.*

Just like kefir and most dairy products, Bulgarian yogurt has wonderful healthy properties and effects.

- ***It is a perfect prevention tool for osteoporosis****, strengthening the bones, teeth, and tissues.*
- ***It is also suitable for diabetics*** *and people with high cholesterol levels.*
- ***It has antibacterial and antifungal properties;***
- ***Supplies with rare types of probiotics*** *that counteract the pathogenic microorganisms in the digestive tract, especially the decay causing ones.*
- ***Prevents from cancer*** *development and supports the immune system;*
- ***Supports the natural weight loss*** – Bulgarian yogurt contains lots of easily digestible proteins and low amounts of carbohydrates. This makes it excellent for achieving a healthy and slender body;
- ***Promotes anti-aging and longevity*** – the famous Russian scientist and founder of the modern immunology, Ilya Metchnikoff, found one of the main reasons people develop illnesses and age faster - intestinal auto-intoxication. On the other hand, he

found that the probiotics in the Bulgarian yogurt tend to inhibit the growth of the colon bacteria that stimulate this auto-intoxication. As a result, Bulgarians and the people from the Russian Steppes, consuming large amounts of traditional yogurt and kefir, have longer and healthier lives.

- ***Heals many gastrointestinal issues, including severe diarrhea.*** Here is an interesting historical fact: the French king Francis I of France was suffering from a serious case of life threatening diarrhea leading to extreme dehydration. Thankfully, he was administrated a special diet consisting of regular consumption of traditional Bulgarian yogurt and the illness was cured. Since then, Bulgarian yogurt gained a lot of popularity throughout Europe. Now it has its loyal fans all the way to Japan!

How to make Bulgarian yogurt at home?

The process is very simple and can be done easily with the needed ingredients, some time, patience, and perfect hygiene. The main thing you will need is fresh high quality milk. It can be cow, goat, sheep, even buffalo. The plant based types of milk will not do for obvious reasons. So, this homemade product is not suitable for strict vegans.

The other essential ingredient is the yeast. You need the special Bulgarian bacterial cultures that cause the yogurt's distinct flavor, taste, and health benefits. As we discussed earlier, Lactobacillus Bulgaricus cannot be found and supported outside Bulgaria, but that does not mean you cannot get it. Now that the fame of Bulgarian yogurt is spreading around the world, you can find lots of companies that provide special starter packs designed to assist you with your own homemade sour milk production. The important thing to remember is that you cannot use the same yeast more than once. In Bulgaria, where this special bacterium grows naturally, you can take a portion of the ready-made yogurt and use it as yeast for the next batch. Unfortunately, outside our region this is not possible. Keep that in mind.

Here I will describe the simplest method in which you don't need a special yogurt maker. If you have one, perfect! You can use it and save yourself some effort.

First, put the milk in a metal pot and heat it. When it just starts to boil take it off the heat and place the lid on top and let it sit for 10-15 minutes. The goal is to reach a temperature of 44-45 degrees C (111-113 degrees F). Remember to use a clean sterilized kitchen thermometer to avoid infiltrating the milk. Now it is time to add the yeast. If you have genuine Bulgarian yogurt, mix 2 Tbsps. of it for each liter (4 cups) of milk. If you have 2 liters milk (8 cups), add 4 Tbsps. yogurt yeast, and so on. Place the yeast in another bowl and add some of the milk in it. Stir the mixture well until it becomes fully homogenous. Add this mixture to the remaining milk and stir well. If you are using a starter pack, follow the instructions and ratios of the product.

Pour the leavened milk in dry and clean glass jars and seal them immediately.

Now it's time for the fermentation. You need to place the jars in a warm place with the perfect temperature (44-45 deg. C/ 111-113 deg. F). If you don't have a yogurt maker, you can place the jars in the oven – just switch on only the convection oven at about 30 deg. C/ 86 F. This will keep a steady temperature without burning the yogurt. If you live in a hot country, you can simply place the jars in a warm and sunny spot. In several hours, the milk should have coagulated and turned into sour yogurt. You can place it in the fridge and consume it on the very next day.

The best thing about this yogurt is that you can use it in various ways – as a dessert mixed with fruits, in your healthy immune boosting recipes, or as an addition to the main meal. Here is a quick healthy breakfast you can prepare fast and support your natural defense system!

Probiotic Fiber Breakfast Recipe

Ingredients:

2 Tbsps. **rye flakes**

2 Tbsps. **barley flakes**

2 Tbsps. **einkorn or emmer**

2 Tbsps. **seed mixture** (sunflower seeds, Golden flax seed, sesame, poppy seeds, etc.)

1 Tbsp. **raw organic honey**

400 grams (1 1/2 cups) **Bulgarian homemade yogurt**

1 cup **pure boiling water**

Directions:

Wash the einkorn (or emmer) grains. Place them in a bowl and pour the hot water in it. In another bowl mix the yogurt, the rye and barley flakes and the seed mixture. Stir well and leave it overnight.

In the morning strain the grains, but do not throw away the water. You can drink it on an empty stomach – it is full of beneficial substances. Add the grains and the honey to the yogurt mixture and stir well. When the honey is fully dissolved, the breakfast is ready! It will supply with lots of probiotics, simple carbohydrates, proteins, energy, and fiber.

Pickles

Homemade pickles using different kinds of bio organic produce can have a significant beneficial effect on our health and immunity. If prepared correctly, with the right ingredients, we can make a wonderful probiotic appetizer and stimulate the growth of the good colon bacteria.

Pickled vegetables are proven to have numerous benefits for the human body:

- ***They speed up the metabolism.*** As a result of the fermentation, the pickles contain lots of enzymes that boost the metabolic processes and fight obesity;
- ***Improve the digestion.*** The enzymes, we spoke of, are extremely beneficial for the gastrointestinal tract, soothing various digestive problems, even ulcers and arthritis.
- ***Have anti-aging effect.*** The health of the colon bacteria is tightly connected to our overall condition, and especially our skin and appearance. When our bodies are full of toxins, have low immunity, the first place you can see this condition is the skin. Skin rashes appear, the derma looks darker, dryer and more susceptible to wrinkles. That is why taking pickled vegetables regularly may brighten the skin and slow down the aging process.
- ***Builds the natural immunity.*** How the heck pickled vegetables boost our natural defense

system? Well, the beneficial colon bacteria love fermented foods. By giving them what they need, we keep them healthy, stimulate their growth, and thus, we sustain our own wellbeing. Taking pickles is extremely beneficial when fighting stubborn infections (like Candida), colds and the flu.

How to prepare your own healthy pickles (without artificial preservatives, and other chemicals)?

Here I will share with you some simple recipes you can try at home and build your natural immunity. We will be using the process of "wild fermentation" to reap the full benefits of the pickled produce. Wild fermentation means that we will let the veggies start the fermenting process without any external agents, like vinegar or yeast. That is how we will create the ultimate healthy probiotic appetizer. Let's begin!

Our first pickles recipe will be cabbage (sauerkraut), because it is the easiest. Once you nail it, you can start making experiments on your own and add more vegetables.

Fast Homemade Sauerkraut

Ingredients:
Cabbage
Salt – sea or Himalayan
Clean **water**
Celery (optional)
Glass jars
Gauze
Clean **heavy object** (to fit in the jars)

Directions:

Choose a cabbage that is pure and not treated with nitrates, pesticides, or other harmful agents. These chemicals are harmful for our bodies and they will slow down (or even stop) the fermentation process.

Next, remove the outer leaves and cut the cabbage in strips. Sprinkle with salt thoroughly and mix them well. We need the cabbage to be well salted. The strips will become slightly softer and the salt will start to dissolve in the vegetable juice. Place the salty cabbage strips in the jars. Try to put as much cabbage as possible and leave as little air as possible. Do NOT add any water at this point! Place gauze on top of the jar and leave it for about 24 hours. The cabbage will start to bleed, which will begin the fermentation process. When the time is up, see if the vegetable juice is enough to submerse the cabbage. If not, add some salty water (2 Tbsps. salt for each liter (4 cups) pure water). Another option is fresh celery juice - it is naturally salty. Now place the heavy object on top of the cabbage. The goal is to keep the vegetables fully submersed at all time. Otherwise, it will start to get moldy. Place the gauze once again and let the jar sit for about 3 days. The duration of the fermentation depends on the temperature of the room. The warmer it is, the faster it will become sour. But the general rule is about 3 days. If the cabbage is not sour enough, you can leave it for one more day until you like the taste of the pickles. When you decide to stop the fermentation, just seal the jar and place it in the fridge. Remember to remove the heavy object from the sauerkraut, we don't need it anymore.

Since we don't use any artificial preservatives in this recipe, the pickles will be edible for up to 3 weeks after preparation.

Colorful Homemade Pickles (Turshi)

Ingredients:
Cauliflower
Carrots
Green tomatoes
Celery stalks
Red peppers
Pure **water**
Sea or Himalayan **salt**
Large **glass jar**
Gauze

Directions:

The quantities of the raw vegetables will depend on your goals and preferences. Wash them thoroughly and cut them in medium pieces. Place them in a large glass jar as tight as possible. Do not fill the whole jar to the top. We need to leave some space for the brine.

Place the water in a metal pot and heat it. For every 1 liter (4 cups) water add 1 Tbsp. salt. Stir until the salt is fully dissolved. Take it off the heat and let it cool off. Pour the salty solution in the jar and submerse the veggies completely. Otherwise, they might get moldy. Place the gauze on top instead of the lid and leave the jar at room temperature. The fermentation process will last from 5 to 7 days. It depends on the temperature of the room and how sour you wish to make the pickles. For extra safety measures, you can place the jar in a plate – the fermentation process will cause the veggies to bulk up and the brine may overflow.

When the pickled vegetables are ready (you like their sour taste), you can seal the jar and put it in the fridge. Remember that the longer you leave the pickles to ferment, the sourer the taste will be. So, taste it every day until you like its flavor.

The product will be edible for up to 3 weeks in the fridge.

Adaptogens and Immunity

"Your body is a temple, but only if you treat it as one."
~Astrid Alauda

When talking about natural strong immunity we must mention the adaptogens. As the name implies, the adaptogens are substances that help our bodies adjust and counteract stress in a healthy way. There is a direct link between our abilities to manage stress and immunity. As I mentioned before, if we experience pressure on a daily basis, our immunity weakens. On the other hand, if we are able to process the stressful conditions, our bodies are strong and healthy. Adaptogens can help us in both ways – boost our immunity and help us de-stress. That is why they are so important and should be an integral part of a healthy lifestyle. Thankfully, Mother Nature never ceases to supply us with beneficial nutrients, and adaptogens are no exception.

Benefits of adaptogens

The adaptogenic substances are known for their libido enhancing properties (for men and women). They are excellent reproductive hormone secretion stimulators. If you have any issues in this area, these plants and animal products can make a huge difference!

The testicles and ovaries are not the only organs benefitting from these immune boosters. All glands of the human endocrine system are tightly connected. And imbalance in one area affects the whole. For example, problems with the thyroid can lead to reproductive hormone imbalances, and vice versa. Another example is the development of osteoporosis. The link between female hormones secretion and bone density has been proven. And adaptogens come to the rescue once again. They regulate the hormone synthesis, stimulate the proper metabolism, and prevent from various age related ailments.

Feel free to add these special products during the changes of the seasons (especially during Spring, Autumn and Winter), after intense workouts and trainings, in cases of very high or low temperatures and temperature fluctuations, thirst and hunger, low oxygen levels, radiations, etc. All extreme circumstances that require our bodies to adapt and survive.

So, adaptogens are indispensable for supporting the whole endocrine system (the connection between the hypothalamus, pituitary, and adrenal glands), boosting the immune system, supporting a healthy libido, and protecting the nervous system from stress overload. Adaptogens are also known to lower the negative effect from harsh chemical medications and chemotherapy; increase the glucose tolerance (prevent from Diabetes development); help heal and lower the risk of infertility in both sexes; soothe the menopause discomforts; support the immunity in cases of invasive operations and lower the risks of complications; stimulate the tissue regeneration and promote anti-aging; counteract the chronic fatigue syndrome, and many more.

Here are some of the most popular and powerful natural adaptogens you can use to boost your immunity, support the nervous system, and help your body adapt to various stress sources:

Ashwagandha (Withania somnifera)

This is a potent healing and boosting plant which comes from the East, mostly India. It is lavishly used in the traditional natural Indian naturopathy – Ayurveda as an immune booster and stress reliever. But ashwagandha offers much more – it holds numerous health benefits for the whole body, organs and systems. Here are some of its major proven benefits:

- ***Decreases the levels of stress hormones*** *(such as cortisol) and* ***fights the adrenal fatigue.*** It is a wonderful natural additive for fighting daily stress.
- ***Protects the thyroid*** – ashwagandha balances the whole endocrine system of the body and the secretion of all hormones, including the thyroid. Medical experiments show that in only 20 days of taking this plant, the production of the essential thyroid hormones T3 and T4 is significantly boosted. The good news is that ashwagandha is suitable for people with both hypo- and hyperthyroidism, but remember to consult with your physician first!
- ***Stimulates the brain activity and fights depression*** – we talked about the decrease of the stress hormone cortisol by taking this magical Indian herb. But what about the "happy" hormones, like serotonin? Ashwagandha gets you covered! It is an excellent mood booster, sharpening our focus and elevates our spirit!
- *Withania somnifera (also called Indian Ginseng) is* ***perfect for preventing and relieving diabetes and high cholesterol levels.*** Ashwagandha has been proven to stimulate the insulin secretion and

to boost the natural insulin sensitivity, which leads to lowering the blood sugar level. Another good result is that it lowers the levels of the triglycerides and subsequently – the "bad" LDL cholesterol.

- ***Fights impotence and improves the sperm count.*** Most adaptogens are known for their libido and potency boosting properties. This Indian herb is not an exception. The logic behind this is the direct relation between stress and potency. Too much daily stress combined with poor diet and no physical activity results in low sperm count and decreased mobility of the semen. With some positive changes and ashwagandha, many couples have finally managed to conceive their first child!
- ***Indispensable for all athletes*** – being a professional sports person means a lot of dedicated physical work, which means regular stress to the body. It needs to adapt and recover fast and to extend its stress tolerance. What better natural way to achieve this than with adaptogens? Ashwagandha is known to balance the adrenal hormones and quickly recover the sore muscles from the extensive training.
- ***Prevents and fights serious diseases like cancer.*** Now we know the relation between the immune system and cancer. As you may have already learned, every single day thousands of cancer cells are being created. And the job of our immune system is to eliminate them and suppress their growth and further development. This is why adaptogens like aswagandha are so valuable these

days. They could be the key to eradicating this modern plague!

How to take it?

Withania somnifera is one really strong herb and it should be taken with caution and responsibility. Consult with your physician or naturopath to discuss the proper doses for you and remember to follow the guidelines of the product. Take brakes after each healing course with this herb.

Tribulus (Tribulus terrestris)

This is a little known annual plant, which has distinct adaptogenic properties. It is mostly found in Southern Europe and Asia, but in today's global market, Tribulus extracts can be acquired almost everywhere. This herb, usually considered as plain weed, contains various bioactive substances that affect beneficially the human body. That is why Tribulus is frequently used in traditional Chinese and Indian (Ayurveda) medicine for the treatment of many ailments and conditions, such as eyesight problems, edemas, cardiovascular diseases, high blood pressure, etc. But the herb is mostly known for its excellent effect on the endocrine system, especially the reproductive segment. In men, the plant is considered to increase the luteinizing hormone in the testicles which is responsible for the testosterone production. And the good news is that in women, the herb does not increase the secretion of testosterone, but gently balances the female hormonal system. This means that Tribulus can be safely used by both men and women. Let's take a quick look at some of the most potent health effects of this plant (also called Devil's-thorn).

- *Tribulus* ***helps people with extremely low appetite****, and can be a valuable asset when dealing with anorexia.*
- *It can be used as a* ***natural aphrodisiac****, especially for men.*
- *It* ***lowers the blood pressure and the cholesterol levels****, and regulates the heart rhythm (excellent for cases of arrhythmia).*
- *Counteracts the development of prostatic hyperplasia (****enlarged prostate****).*
- *Tribulus has* ***anti-inflammatory effects.***
- ***Helps with the proper digestion*** *of carbohydrates and prevents from blood sugar surges.*
- *The herb also has some* ***distinct analgesic properties.***
- ***Prevents from cataract development*** *(walleye).*
- *Devil's-thorn is* ***excellent for detoxing the liver and kidneys****, especially from heavy metals like Cadmium and Mercury. It also stimulates the production and the recovery of the liver enzymes.*
- *Tribulus has a* ***gentle diuretic effect and antibacterial and antifungal properties****, which make it perfect for treatment of various urinary conditions.*
- *The herb* ***stimulates the immunity, the metabolism, and the proper blood circulation****.*

How to take Tribulus?

First, consult with your physician before self-medicating with this plant. Next, if you decide to go for Tribulus supplements, follow the guidelines of your doctor and the dosages in the product's leaflet.

If you choose the herbal infusion, you can use the following scheme:

Take 1 liter (4 cups) pure water and bring it to boil. Add 5 Tbsps. of the plant and let it simmer for an hour. Strain the infusion and add more water to reach the initial amount (4 cups). Pour the tea in a glass bottle, seal it and place it in the fridge for 24 hours.

The first day of the treatment: take 3 Tbsps. 3 times a day after a meal.

The second day: take 4 Tbsps. 3 times a day after a meal.

From day three to the end of the infusion: 5 Tbsps. 3 times a day.

Tribulus is not suitable for pregnant women, and people with severe gastrointestinal inflammations, acute gastritis, and for small children!

Rhodiola (Rhodiola Rosea)

Rhodiola is a special plant with powerful adaptogenic properties. Usually, it can be found in the cold Northern parts of the world – Siberia, Northern China, Iceland, etc. And its placement is in perfect harmony with its boosting effects on the body. The extract from Rhodiola helps our bodies adapt and withstand various stressful conditions, such as cold/hot weather, infections, extensive physical exercises, even high altitudes. This precious plant is part of the traditional naturopathic medicine of the northern cultures – the Russians, Norwegians, Mongols, Chinese, etc. It is said that the mighty Vikings used Rhodiola to keep themselves in excellent physical and mental shape and to boost their stamina. In the central Asian cultures, Rhodiola is valued as one of the best natural remedies for colds and the flu. And the Mongols use it even to treat serious ailments like tuberculosis and cancer.

Let's see why all these though northern nations use and honor Rhodia so much:

- *Rhoriola can be used to* ***counteract hypotension*** *(low blood pressure), especially in the initial stages.*
- *As a typical example of an adaptogen, this plant* ***fights depression, anxiety, moodiness, and elevates the emotional state****.*
- *It can be used to* ***boost the stamina, fight chronic fatigue and migraines*** *related to this condition.*
- *Rhodiola is the perfect natural assistant to athletes, both professional and dilettantes. It* ***supports the recovery of the muscles and ligaments*** *after extensive and regular physical strain.*
- *This precious plant* ***stimulates the brain activity and boosts our ability to focus****, also prevents from memory loss. It can be used even by people engaged in constant mental work and pressure.*
- *Rhodiola* ***contains lots of antioxidants and cancer cell killing agents****. It also boosts our natural immunity and helps our bodies deal with all malevolent agents on its own. Many researches show that the herb prolongs the lifespan of animals suffering from different types of cancer.*

- ***Rhodiola is a powerful detoxifier** – it has been proven effective to expel various toxins from the body and especially from our most important detoxing power plant – the liver.*
- *Helps us **soothe the symptoms of altitude sickness** – nausea, flatulence, fatigue, dizziness, weakness, swelling, etc.*
- ***Protects from the negative effects of chemotherapy**, especially the liver.*
- *The herb also **lowers the blood sugar level, speeds the metabolism** and promotes a healthy weight loss, **supports the thyroid function** (helps people with hypothyroidism), and works as a powerful aphrodisiac for both men and women.*

How to take Rhodiola?

First of all, just let me remind you that adaptogens are very potent plants and should be taken with responsibility and after a consultation with a physician or a certified herbalist. ***The plant is not suitable for small children and pregnant/breastfeeding women.***

Rhodiola can usually be found in the form of tinctures and the dosage is 30 drops 3 times a day. Try to take the last dosage not later than the early afternoon – Rhodiola is a powerful toner and can cause insomnia if taken in the evening. Or simply follow the guidelines of your doctor or the product's leaflet.

Most adaptogens have similar beneficial effects on our bodies. And Mother Nature gave us plenty of choices for us to pick from. Apart from Aswaganda, Tribulus and Rhodiola, there are countless more adaptogens we can include in our healthy and healing routines: **apitherapeutic products** (Gelee Royal, Bee pollen – we will pay extra attention to bee products in the next chapter), **Pantocrine, Panax ginseng, Eleutherococcus senticosus, Leuzea carthamoides, Shizandra chinesis, Potentilla reptans, Verbena off, Maca, Muira Puama (Ptychopetalum olacoides), Reishi mushrooms**, etc.

Take a look at some yummy adaptogenic recipes!

Ashwagandha Immune Boosting Recipe

Ingredients:

1 Tbsp. ground **flax seeds**
1 **lemon**
2 cm (~1 inch) **ginger root**
1 liter (~4 cups) **pure water**
1 tsp. **lecithin granules**
1/4 tsp. **purple maize powder**
1/4 tsp. **ashwagandha powder**

Directions:

Soak the ground flax seeds in some pure water in the evening. Let it sit overnight so that it forms its special healing mucus-like substance. Squeeze the juice out of the lemon, peel and cut the ginger root in pieces. Place all ingredients in a blender and mix until it is fully homogenous. The recipe is for 4 servings.

Maca Smoothie

Ingredients:
6 fresh **strawberries**
1 **banana**
1-2 Tbsps. **Maca powder**

Directions:
Place all ingredients in a blender and stir until the consistency is fully homogenous. In the summer, you can add some ice cubes to make the smoothie more refreshing and energizing.

Healthy Chocolate Maca Cookies

Ingredients:
1/4 cup **almond milk**
2 Tbsps. **coconut butter**
1 Tbsp. **vanilla extract**
1 cup **coconut sugar** or grade B **maple syrup**
1 1/2 cup **wholegrain flour**
1 Tbsp. **Maca powder**
1/2 Tbsp. **baking soda**
1 Tbsp. **baking powder**
1/2 Tbsp. sea or Himalayan **salt** (ground)
1/2 cup bio dark natural **chocolate chips**

Directions:
Start heating the oven beforehand to 180 degrees Celsius (~350 F). When the cookies are ready for baking, the oven needs to be hot.

In a large bowl mix the flour, Maca powder, baking soda, baking powder, and the salt. Melt the coconut butter and mix it with the almond milk. Add the liquid mixture to the bowl with the dry ingredients and start stirring until you reach the consistency of sticky dough.

Take a suitable baking pan and cover it with oiled baking paper. Start scooping from the dough, form small balls, and place them in the baking pan. Press the balls gently to flatten them a little bit in order for them to be easily baked. Bake the cookies for about 16 minutes until they form a golden brown crust.

Maca Pudding

Ingredients:

2 Tbsps. **Chia seeds**

1 Tbsp. **cocoa powder**

1 Tbsp. **Maca powder**

1 cup **almond milk**

Some healthy **sugar** – coconut sugar, agave syrup, maple syrup, etc.

Directions:

Mix the almond milk and the Chia seeds in a blender. Be careful not to let any dry Chia lumps remain in the mix. Add the cocoa, Maca and the sugar and blend until full homogeneousness.

Pour the mixture in a suitable glass container with a lid and place it in the fridge for 8 hours. Serve cold and enjoy

Apitherapy for the Immune System

"Life is not merely to be alive, but to be well."
~Marcus Valerius Martial

Apitherapy is a special type of the natural healing system. It is focused on the wonderful and powerful nourishing, healing, and boosting properties of bee products. It can be divided into several types, as well, depending on the bee product we would like to use: honey treatment, Gelee Royal treatment, pollen therapy, apitoxin therapy, propolis therapy, and beewax therapy. For the purpose of boosting our natural immunity we will concentrate on those bee products that have the most prominent strengthening effects. Namely:

Honey

In book 1 of the series, we talked a lot about all the wonderful benefits of raw (unpasteurized) organic honey. It is not just a healthy white sugar alternative, but it is a powerful immune booster on its own. As you can see in this volume, honey is an integral part of most detoxing, healing, and strengthening recipes. Beside its sweet taste, honey is packed with nutrients, enzymes, minerals, microelements, etc. It has strong antimicrobial, anti-viral, anti-cancer, and anti-fungal effects without harming our bodies and beneficial colon bacteria. For boosting your immunity, prepare some of the recipes in this book, or take a tablespoon of the divine nectar daily on an empty stomach. Remember not to heat the honey above body temperature.

In the chapters below you will see plenty of immune boosting recipes with honey. But for now, you can take a look at this precious one – excellent for preventing and soothing cardiovascular issues:

Geranium Immune Booster and Toner

Ingredients:
200 grams (~1 cup) raw **organic honey**
3-4 bio **lemons**
20 fresh **Geranium leaves**
30 raw **almonds or walnuts**

Directions:

Soak the nuts the night before in some pure water. Wash them thoroughly the next day. Squeeze the lemons, but do not throw away the zest. Next, wash the Geranium leaves and put them in a kitchen chopper or food processor. Add the lemon juice, the lemon zest, and the nuts. Mince the ingredients well. Put the mixture in a glass jar and add the honey. Stir until everything is fully blended. Seal it and store in the fridge.

Take 1 Tbsp. every morning on an empty stomach 30 minutes before breakfast.

Why Geranium?

Geranium is usually considered to be a house plant with nice refreshing aroma. But it holds lots of health benefits. It is no wonder that in most Slavic nations it is called "health giver". It is frequently used in our traditional naturopathic medicine for various conditions, such as diarrhea, arrhythmia, hypertension, all kinds of hemorrhages (including uterine), rheumatism, skin infections, wounds, fatigue, anxiety, nervous tension, insomnia, arthritis, burns, coughs, flu, laryngitis, and even diabetes.

Important note: Geranium contains insulin-like substances that may quickly lower the blood sugar level. In case you have any related health conditions (or any other serious chronic illness), do not hesitate to consult with your physician before applying this recipe.

Propolis

This is the bee products' heavy artillery when it comes to fighting germs and boosting the immunity. Propolis is the natural defense system of the bee hive – it protects it from bacteria, viruses, and fungi. Thankfully, it has the same protective effects on our system as well. Take a look at the countless benefits of propolis regular use:

- *Propolis is one of the best natural (without side effects) cures for* ***gastrointestinal issues like gastritis and ulcers****.*
- *If used topically, it* ***heals all kinds of skin problems*** *(eczemas, rashes, wounds), hemorrhoids, and varicose veins, preventing from intravascular coagulation. You can even use it as a disinfecting and healing treatment for the oral cavity, especially for infections and receding gums.*
- *It has strong* ***antibacterial and bacteriostatic effects*** *(kills the pathogenic bacteria and stops their growth). The best part is – these effects remain intact even at high temperatures (unlike honey).*
- *Propolis also has* ***powerful anti-fungal properties*** *– it can be applied for fighting germs*

and inflammatory processes in the gastrointestinal tract, the oral cavity, the respiratory system, etc.

- *Its anti-viral effect makes it perfect for* ***preventing and fighting the flu, colds, and even viral herpes****.*
- *Propolis* ***guards our organism from all kinds of unwelcomed guest****, including various types of parasites.*
- *Surprisingly, this bee product also* ***has analgesic effects*** *(works as a mild painkiller). The effect can be observed 5-10 minutes after application.*
- *Propolis is a valuable assistant* ***for people with high blood pressure****.*
- *This natural multilateral product has much more to offer – it is proven to* ***counteract the development of sclerosis and cancer****. It has distinct anabolic, antispasmodic, anti-oxidant, anti-radiation, and detoxing effects.*
- *And last, but not least – it is* ***one of the post powerful natural immune boosters*** *known to man.*

As you can see, propolis is definitely something any household should have in their medicinal cabinet. ***With one exception – any allergies of bee products. In this case, you should avoid propolis and its derivatives.***

For the purpose of strengthening the immune system, we will use propolis tincture – it is an alcohol solution of propolis. You can buy it directly from the pharmacy or prepare it on your own. The procedure is very simple: take 40 grams (~2 1/2 Tbsps.) propolis and 100 ml (~3.38 o.z.) alcohol (vodka, brandy, etc.). Grate the propolis and mix it with the liquor in a glass jar. Seal it and place it in a dark and cool place. Shake the mixture several times a day. In about a week, the tincture should be ready. Strain it with fine cheesecloth and put the alcohol infusion in a tightly sealed jar or bottle. It will keep its healing properties for up to 3 years.

How to take propolis tincture for boosting the immunity?

If you have prepared your tincture at home, you will need a pipette. Take 30 drops of the tincture, mix it with some pure water, and take the mixture at least 30 minutes before a meal 3 times a day. The prevention course can last about 30 days. Then you can take a break a couple of weeks and repeat the process.

For those who cannot take alcohol in any form and for children, you can apply the water infusion instead. Consult with your pediatrician before applying this on your kids. ***The product is not suitable for children below 3 years of age.***

Here is how to prepare the water infusion.

Take 100 grams (~7 Tbsps.) grated propolis and 100 ml (~3.38 o.z.) distilled water. Place the ingredients in a double boiler and put it on low heat. Stir the mixture for several hours. Filter it with a strainer and fine cheesecloth. The administration is the same as the tincture – 30 drops 3 times a day on an empty stomach.

Always make an allergy test before applying any new bee products! For example, take one drop of the propolis tincture and mix it with some water. Drink and pay attention to any peculiar sensations – itching, swelling, low blood pressure, etc. If that is the case, seek medical attention immediately and cease taking the bee product.

Here is a nice immune boosting recipe with Propolis.

Propolis & Citrus Shake

Ingredients:
2 **oranges**
2 **tangerines**
1 **mango**
200 ml (~1 cup) Greek or **Bulgarian yogurt**
1/3 tsp. **propolis tincture**
Some **pure water**
1 tsp. **honey** (optional)

Directions:

Peel the fruits and remove all kernels and seeds. Place all ingredients in a blender and stir until everything is fully homogenous. You can regulate the consistency of the drink by changing the quantity of the water. If you like your shake to be sweeter, add the honey and stir until it dissolves.

Take this immune boosting beverage on an empty stomach 40 minutes to an hour before a meal, preferably in the morning.

Gelee Royal

Gelee Royal is another excellent bee product we can use for prevention of all kinds of ailments, for healing, and boosting our natural defense system. It is extremely nutritious – full of vitamins, minerals, microelements, and active substances that support our organism and all of its organs and systems. Here is why I pay attention to this natural gold mine:

- *Gelee Royal stimulates the metabolism;*
- *Lowers the cholesterol levels;*
- *Supports the blood generating process;*
- *Regulates and stimulates the glands;*
- *Works as a natural antibiotic and anti-viral agent (without harming the colon bacteria);*
- *Has a distinct anti-aging effect;*
- *It has anti-inflammatory and immune modulating effects. This means that Gelee Royal is excellent even for people with overactive immune system (auto-immune health conditions), for example Graves' disease.*
- *Supports the growth of the neurons, and thus – helps our nervous system regenerate;*
- *Stimulates the growth of stem cells;*
- *Boosts the immune system and helps us fight all kinds of bacteria, fungi, viruses, and diseases, like cancer.*

How to take Gelee Royal?

It depends on the type of product you are using – gel, powder, tablets, capsules, etc. Just follow the guidelines in the leaflet or your doctor's prescription.

If you have some Gelee Royal gel, you can apply this precious recipe:

Potent Immunity Gelee Royal Recipe

Ingredients:

250 grams (~1 cup) **dry apricots**
250 grams (~1 cup) **raw walnuts**
250 grams (~1 cup) **raisins**
2 **lemons**
1 kilo (~ 4 cups) raw **organic honey**
10 grams (2 tsps.) **Gelee Royal**

Directions:

The dry fruits should not be processed with chemicals and should not contain additional sugar. First, soak the walnuts overnight and wash them well the next day. Take the dry apricots and cut them in pieces. Wash the lemons and cut them as well, remove all seeds. Place the fruits and nuts in a food processor or a chopper and mince them well. Put the mixture in a glass jar and add the bee products. Stir well until everything is fully homogenous. Seal the jar and store in the fridge.

Take 1 Tbsp. 2 times a day (morning and evening) on an empty stomach.

For small children, the dose is 1 tsp. 2 times a day.

Make sure you or your kids do not have any bee product allergies and consult with your physician/pediatrician before applying this recipe.

Bee Pollen

Bee pollen is basically the male germ-cells of the flowering plants. The bees collect this precious powder and store it in the honeycombs. There the bees cover it with honey and the pollen undergoes a fermentation process. That is how it becomes more nutritious and beneficial – full of **essential amino acids** (arginine, isoleucine, histidine, leucine, lysine, methionine, phenylalanine, threonine, Tryptophan, valine, alanine, glycine, asparagine, glutamine, serine, proline, tyrosine, cystine, cysteine), **enzymes, hormones, carbohydrates** (glucose, fructose, sucrose, arabinose, ribose, galactose, raffinose, stachyose, xylose, dextrin, starch, cellulose and lactose), **minerals and microelements** (Potassium, Magnesium, Titanium, Silver, Zinc, Copper, Chromium, Vanadium, Cobalt, Molybdenum, Nickel, Gallium, Zirconium, Manganese, Phosphorus, Silicon, Calcium, Iron, Aluminum, Barium), **vitamins** (C, B1, B2, B5, B6, B8, E, provitamin A, folic acid, biotin, tocopherol), **natural safe antibiotics, biologically active substances, lipids, aromatics and pigments**, etc. Bee pollen is one of the best natural food supplements we can have on our table – it contains everything our organism needs to be healthy and vibrant.

As you can see bee pollen is packed with nutrients and active substances. And these beneficial chemicals have numerous positive healing, preventive, and restoring effects on our bodies. It is the ultimate healthy supplement! Just take a look:

- *Bee pollen* ***helps building our bone system*** *– excellent for children (without bee product allergies) and prevention of osteoporosis development;*

- *Fights* ***impotence and frigidity*** *due to its high amounts of vitamin E;*
- ***Strengthens the blood vessels****, blood cells, the heart, and the overall cardiovascular system;*
- ***Regulates the metabolism*** *and helps with natural safe weight loss;*
- *The Selenium* ***prevents from Alzheimer's disease*** *and gently detoxes the body, even from heavy metals;*
- *Powerful assistant in* **counteracting diabetes** *– stimulates the production of insulin;*
- *The Iodine in bee pollen is excellent for* ***prevention from thyroid issues;***
- ***Heals and soothes various gastrointestinal conditions*** *– colitis, IBS, flatulence, etc.*
- ***Excellent addition to anemia treatments*** *due to the containing Iron;*
- ***Lowers the cholesterol level*** *and fights atherosclerosis;*
- ***Stimulates the tissue regeneration*** *and the proper blood flow, so it has a distinct anti-aging effect;*
- *Powerful addition to* ***managing chronic fatigue, allergies and respiratory problems;***
- ***Fights depression and anxiety;***
- ***Excellent for physically active people*** *and those recovering from serious illnesses or surgeries. Apply only after consulting with your physician first!*
- *And, of course,* **helps the immune system** *and fights bacteria, germs, viruses, fungi, etc.*

The daily doses are:
For adults – 1 Tbsp.
Children from 3 to 5 years old – 1-2 tsps.
Children from 6 to 12 years old – 2-3 tsps.
Consult with your pediatrician first!
Important note: in order for the bee pollen to do its magic properly, it needs to be dissolved first. The ideal substance is something sour and acid, like the Bulgarian yogurt or citrus juice. Mix it with the pollen the night before and let it sit overnight to fully dissolve. You can add some raw honey to sweeten the mixture.
Do not forget to take your free pdf recipe book "10 Powerful Immune Boosting Recipes"! There you will find some very potent formulas using the amazing bee pollen and Gelee Royal!

Here is another cool recipe you can try:

Fig Smoothie

Ingredients:
180 ml (6 o.z.) **almond milk**
1 ripe **banana**
20 **grapes**
6 **figs**
1/2 tsp. **raw honey**
1 Tbsp. **vanilla extract**
1 1/2 Tbsp. **bee pollen**
A pinch of **Himalayan salt** (ground)

Directions:

Place the almond milk, the banana, 18 grapes, 5 1/2 figs, the honey, vanilla extract and 1 tsp. bee pollen in a blender. Mince the mixture until it is fully homogenous. Pour it in a cup and decorate with the remaining 2 grapes, 1/2 fig, and 1/2 Tbsp. bee pollen.

Boosting the Immune System with Homeopathy

"And in homeopathy the methods are similar to those of Love. Until now, all people were allopathic. Now it is time to go to homeopathy – from large to low doses."

~Peter Dunov (Beinsa Duno)

The classical Homeopathy and its variations (Shussler salts, Bach flowers) can be extremely valuable when stimulating our natural defense system and prevention of all kinds of diseases.

There are countless homeopathic remedies, specially designed for safely boosting the immune system, such as:

- **Oscillococcinum** – this is probably the most popular Homeopathic remedy in the world. It is a combined remedy that has been proven to be effective for prevention and treatment of the flu. For preparation during the flu season and boosting our immunity, you can take 1 dose weekly from Fall and during the whole flu season.
- **Influenzinum 15CH** – this is a mono homeopathic remedy specially designed for flu prevention (it is produced from a flu vaccine). Take 10 granules weekly during the flu season.
- **Echinacea angustifolia 5CH** – the plant Echinacea is a proven immune booster all around the world. But we can use it in the form of a homeopathic remedy as well. Some medical specialists state that the homeopathic form is even

more effective. There is no harm in applying it anyway. So, for preventive purposes take 5 granules 2 times a day. This product is most effective during its first 14 days of application. So, change the immune boosting remedy every 2 weeks for best results.

- **Engystol** – this is another combined homeopathic immune booster, which had proven its effectiveness through various experiments and researches. It contains two main ingredients that affect beneficially our defense system, stimulating the phagocytosis and the lymphocytes production. It works wonderfully on both adults and children. For boosting the immunity and prevention, the dose for adults and kids older than 3 is 1 tablet 3 times a day. For smaller children – half a tablet 3 times a day.
- **Esberitox** – it contains four main homeopathic remedies combined in perfect synergy. Take 1 tablet 3 times a day to stimulate your natural defense system and prevent from various diseases.
- **Influcid** – this is a powerful combined remedy consisting of 6 homeopathic ingredients. Influcid has been proven very effective, especially against acute viral infections. For prevention take 2 tablets 2 times a day.
- **Immunokind** - a special immune booster for kids. The dose is 1 tablet 3 times a day. If the child is too small to let the remedy melt in their mouth, dissolve the tablets in some pure water.

Remember, homeopathic treatment is personal and the best course of action, of course, is to consult with a certified

Homeopathic specialist. They will prescribe you the best remedies according to your needs, your character, and emotionality. As we talked in book 2, Homeopathy works best when the recipe is personal and prescribed from a skilled specialist. Also consult with your physician or pediatrician in case you have any chronic or acute illnesses, allergies, etc. Homeopathy is considered safe, but keep in mind that there is still a possibility of having allergies to some of the ingredients. ***Diabetics should not take homeopathic remedies before consulting with a doctor – most of these tablets and granules contain some sugar.***

Keep in mind that the homeopathic remedies are different from the regular medications and their administration is peculiar. If you want to take the most out of them, put the tablets/granules under the tongue until they are fully dissolved. This process should be done at least 30 minutes before any meal or drink. If you have just brushed your teeth, had a meal, drank coffee, or smoked a cigarette, etc. wait for at least 40 minutes before taking the remedies. ***You should not have any taste in your mouth – this is crucial for the effectiveness of the treatment.***

Of course there are many things we can do on our own. And beside the homeopathic remedies, listed above, we can also include the powerful Shussler salts. These are also types of natural remedies, using the same homeopathic principles. Here are the top salts you can use to boost your immunity naturally:

Shussler salts

As we have discussed in book 2, the Shussler salts are another excellent type of homeopathic remedies, suitable for soothing and preventing various health ailments. They are also perfect for boosting our immunity in a safe and powerful way. You can apply the following remedies:

- **Shussler salt # 3 (Ferrum phosphoricum D12)**
  It helps with the oxygen transfer in our bodies. It boosts the immunity by stimulating the production of antibodies that attack the viruses in the early stages of the infection. Take 3 tablets in the morning – dissolve them in some warm water or directly in the mouth (let them dissolve slowly). If you want to counteract the flu or a cold, suck 1 tablet every 5 minutes during the first symptoms.
- **Shussler salt # 6 (Kalium sulfuricum D6)**
  This is a perfect immune booster and detoxifier for recovering from an illness and stimulating our defense system. It takes out all waste products accumulated during the healing period. Take 3 tablets in the evening by slowly salivating them in the mouth or dissolve them in some warm water beforehand.
- **Shussler salt # 10 (Natrium sulfuricum D6)**
  This salt is good to be taken in combination with Shussler salt #6 for fully detoxing and recovering from an illness. The administration is the same as Salt #6 – 3 tablets in the evening in some water or directly in the mouth.

- **Shussler salt # 7 (Magnesium phosphoricum D6)**

  As the name implies, this homeopathic salt derives from the mineral Magnesium. It soothes any pains and tension in the nerves and muscles. It helps us relax, sleep better and counteract the seasonal depression and mood swings. Take 3 tablets at noon, dissolved in some warm water or let them slowly disintegrate in the mouth.

Other Powerful Immunity Boosters and Modulators

"Take care of your body. It's the only place you have to live."
~Jim Rohn

Aloe Vera

There are more than 500 types of Aloe and not all of them have healing powers for the human body. Some of them are even poisonous! Here by the term Aloe Vera we will discuss Aloe Barbadensis Miller – the plant among all types of Aloe with holds the most health benefits for us humans.

Aloe is one of the best all-purpose natural substances for us. It has numerous positive effects on our organism and here I will list just the most potent and important ones:

- *Aloe Vera (especially its gel) is one of the best* ***natural laxatives*** *for our gastrointestinal tract without causing any negative side effects.*
- *Supports and stimulates the* ***function of the liver and the digestion****.*
- *It helps us absorb the nutrients of the foods and* ***boosts our metabolism****.*
- *Aloe gently and safely* ***purifies the blood****, strengthens the immunity and invigorates our organism.*
- *This magical healing plant has been proven to be* ***very effective against tumors****, especially colon and ovarian cancer.*

- ***Balances the hormones,*** *soothes all PMS symptoms and even prevents and heals from ovarian cysts.*
- *Aloe Vera also has the power to normalize and* ***lower the high blood sugar levels****, which makes it extremely valuable for people with diabetes.*
- *Aloe is effective against* ***skin issues*** *(eczemas, psoriasis, dermatitis, burns), herpes, and aphthous stomatitis as well.*
- *There are even some extensive researches for the plant's* ***positive effects against AIDS****.*

Why is aloe so special?

The Aloe plant contains 2 chemical compounds which are hard to find - acemannan and allantoin. Acemannan is a special carbohydrate molecule with a protein core. Our organism synthesizes this compound, but only during puberty. After that, we need to supply it with our food. And doing so is highly recommended because Acemannan activates the immune-mediators, such as interleukin 1. With regards to allantoin, we cannot synthesize this chemical on our own. Which is why foods containing this compound are very important for us. Allantoin is a powerful anti-oxidant, which detoxes the cells and supports the natural immunity.

A story of Aloe and skin cancer

I would like to tell you a story, which perfectly shows the power of the Aloe plant. Not long ago I was watching a random video on the web of a passionate gardener. The guy has been planting and growing his own beautiful flowers and medicinal herbs at his home. And many of those plants were Aloes. But one day he noticed a strange mole on his arm, which unfortunately turned out to be a carcinoma. And since he was dealing with this healing plant and he knew how beneficial it was for our bodies, he made an experiment. Every day as he was working in his garden, he would chop a leaf off the Aloes and rubbed its healing gel on the mole. And lo and behold, after some time of regular treatment, the carcinoma disappeared!

Important: let this story work as an example and a showcase of the amazing powers of Aloe. In case you have any serious ailments, consult with your physician and avoid self-medicating and self-treatment without medical assistance or surveillance!

Also keep in mind that Aloe is a very strong healing plant and it has its counter-indications and side effects. The Aloe products are not suitable for people with acute kidney and gastrointestinal issues, during pregnancy, inflammations in the female reproductive system, some heart diseases, tuberculosis, hemorrhoids, allergy to the plant, etc. Consult with a doctor before applying and healing with Aloe.

Healthy healing recipes with Aloe:

Acad. Filatov's[1] Aloe & Wine Recipe for the Liver

Ingredients:
150 grams (~1/2 cup) **Aloe leaves**
250 grams (1 cup) **raw organic honey**
350 ml (1 1/2 cup) **strong wine** (about 17 deg.)

Directions:

You can buy the Aloe Vera leaves or ask from a friend. For this recipe you need fresh Aloe leaves at least 3-4 years old. If you have Aloe Barbadendis Miller at home and you wish to use it for healing purposes, move the plant in a dark place and stop watering it for about a week. This is how it will accumulate more of its precious substances in the leaves and gel.

When you supply the leaves, wash them thoroughly and gently cut their spikes off. Next, place them in a food processor or a chopper and dice them. In a proper glass container put the Aloe puree, the honey and the wine and mix well. The healing recipe is ready!

Take 1 Tbsp. of the mixture half an hour before a meal 3 times a day.

---

[1] *Vladimir Petrovich Filatov is world renowned Russian/Ukrainian ophthalmologist and surgeon. He became famous for his development of tissue therapy, tube flap grafting method, and the introduction of corneal transplantation.*

Acad. Filatov's Aloe Recipe for Stronger Immunity and Better Eyesight

Ingredients:
100 grams (~1/2 cup) **Aloe juice**
500 grams (2 cups) **raw walnuts**
300 grams (1 1/4 cup) **raw organic honey**
3-4 **lemons**

Directions:

Squeeze the juice from the lemons and grind the walnuts. Mix all ingredients in a glass container and stir well.

Take 1 Tbsp. of the mixture 3 times a day on an empty stomach.

If you are using your own plant for the recipe, follow the same rules from the previous recipe. The plant needs to be at least 3 years of age, stop watering it for a week, and then you can cut the leaves. Acad. Filatov even recommends the cut leaves to be placed in the fridge for 10-12 days. According to him, these are the perfect conditions for the Aloe to produce special compounds called "biogenic stimulators", which stimulate the processes in our organism and boost our immunity.

Refreshing and Boosting Aloe Smoothie

Ingredients:
1/4 cup **Aloe juice**
1/2 **apple** (preferably green)
1/2 **cucumber**
1 **kiwi**
1/2 **lemon**
A small piece of **ginger root**
1 Tbsp. ground **flax seeds**
Some **pure water**

Directions:

Place the flax seeds in some pure water the night before. They will bulk up and form their healing mucus-like substance.

On the next day, cut the apple, the cucumber and the kiwi in smaller pieces and place them in a blender. Puree the fruits and then cut the ginger root. Add the ginger to the fruit mix and stir again. Next, squeeze the juice from the lemon and add it in the blender. Put the Aloe juice and the flax seeds in as well and blend all ingredients completely. Enjoy!

Brewer's yeast

Brewer's yeast (or beer yeast) is a product derived from malt and hops. It contains a special culture of beneficial bacteria called Saccharomyces cerevisiae – essential in beer brewing, winemaking and baking. This natural substance, called by the Greeks "sweet mold" or "sugar fungi", is full of valuable nutrients and healthy substances. This makes brewer's yeast extremely beneficial for the human organism and its well-being. Let's take a quick peak of all the goodies in this underrated natural product! Beer yeast is rich in vitamins from the group B – essential for our good health: B1 (Thiamine), B2 (Riboflavin), B3 (Niacin), B5 (Pantothenic acid), B6 (Pyridoxine), B9 (Folic acid), and the ultra-important B12 (Cobalamin). The product also contains lots of minerals and micro elements, such as Calcium, Potassium, Phosphorus, Iron, Copper, Manganese, Zinc, Sodium, etc.

Brewer's yeast is extremely important for all vegetarians, vegans, and active athletes – it supplies us not only with carbohydrates, but also with essential proteins, and fiber. When choosing your brewer's yeast keep in mind the following guidelines:

- *Choose a high quality product from a trusted source;*
- *Check if the yeast contains any GMO ingredients;*
- *Choose pure yeast without any additional unwanted agents, like fillers or binders (bonding substances). These are usually found in lyophilized tablets. That is why the best choice of brewer's yeast is in the form of dried flakes.*
- *Chromium – usually the natural brewer's yeast do not contain Chromium, or at least not in very large quantities. Pay attention if your chosen product contains this mineral or not. This is especially important to people suffering from diabetes, because Chromium has been proven to lower the blood sugar level.*

What are the benefits of natural beer yeast?

Due to its rich content, Saccharomyces cerevisiae has proven its positive effects on our bodies in multiple ways:

- **It boosts the immunity** – beer yeast supports our overall health and well-being and especially the regeneration of the tissues. It works as a probiotic and helps us fight infections and viruses.
- **Speeds the metabolism** – the metabolism is tightly connected to our gastrointestinal tract. As we have learned, beer yeast stimulates the growth of the beneficial colon bacteria, fights infections in the intestines, stimulates the digestion, and even soothes many health conditions in this area (such as diarrhea). And due to its high amounts of fiber, brewer's yeast stimulates the bowel movement and promotes a natural weight loss.
- **Supports the nervous system** – the vitamins of group B are essential for the nerves' health and regeneration. These essential compounds stimulate the transmission of the nervous impulses, increase our abilities to focus, and boost the work of the brain cells.
- **The ultimate beauty supplement** – regular administration of beer yeast helps the condition of our hair, nails and skin. It stimulates the metabolic processes and speeds the regeneration of the tissues. Beer yeast can be used safely both internally and externally as hair/skin masks and beauty treatments.

Do you need any ideas?

Here are some recipes for you to try in incorporating beer yeast in your healthy diet. I know taking supplements seems boring, so take a look at my suggestions to you:

Boosting Brewer's Yeast Smoothie

Ingredients:
1 **banana**
2 **fresh dates** (without the kernels, of course)
2 Tbsps. **sesame tahini**
2 Tbsps. **beer yeast flakes**
1 cup **water**

Directions:
Place all ingredients in the blender and mix until you reach the desired consistency.

This drink is extremely nutritional and it is excellent for nourishing an exhausted body (recovering from physical or mental stress or a disease) and for active athletes.

Vegan Cream Cheese

Ingredients:
Some **nuts** (also can be sprouts)
Some **beer yeast flakes**
garlic
1 lemon
Choose the quantities according to your taste and desired end result.

Directions:
Cut the lemon in large pieces and remove any seeds. Peel the garlic cloves. Place all ingredients in a food processor and blend until you reach a homogenous mixture. You can add some water if the consistency is too dry.

Lentils Pate

Ingredients:
Lentils
Beer yeast flakes
Salt
Pepper
Parsley
Choose the quantities according to your taste and desired end result.

Directions:

Boil the lentils until they are fully cooked. Mix all ingredients in a food processor and stir.

This is an excellent appetizer as a spread for wholegrain bread.

Zucchinis with Brown Rice

Ingredients:

1 1/2 cup **brown rice**
2 medium **zucchinis**
1 clove **garlic**
2 Tbsps. **brewer's yeast flakes**
Some pure **water**
The quantities are for 2 servings.

Directions:

Boil the brown rice in the water on low heat until it's fully cooked. Dice the garlic clove. Cut the zucchinis in slices and stew them with the garlic. Mix the brown rice with the beer yeast and add this mixture to the zucchinis. Stir well and the meal is ready!

Wild garlic tincture

Wild garlic (Allium ursinum) is a little known plant with lots of health benefits. It is considered to be even more potent than the regular garlic. The plant is also called ramsons (or bear's garlic) and it can be used for prevention and treatment of various ailments. It is extremely effective against chronic skin issues (lichens, acne, peeling skin, etc.), viruses, colds, fever, rheumatism and joint pain, gastrointestinal and heart conditions, insomnia, high blood pressure, colon parasites, gout, and more. The fresh leaves and bulbs of the plant can be a powerful natural detoxing remedy, which purifies the blood and restores our well-being.

Important! Bear's garlic is a wild plant and it looks very similar to the Lily of the valley (Convallaria majalis) and the autumn crocus (Colchicum autumnale), which are not edible and could lead to poisoning. If you are not a specialist in wild plants, do not harvest wild garlic on your own. Use only trusted suppliers!

Here is how to make your own wild garlic tincture:

Fill a glass jar or a bottle with washed and diced fresh wild garlic leaves and bulbs. Pour strong liquor (vodka, brandy) to fully cover the plant. Seal the container and put in a warm and sunny place. In 14-21 days the tincture is ready. Strain it with cheesecloth and store in a dark and cool place.

For a detoxing and healing course take 10 drops of the remedy 3 times a day on an empty stomach (30 minutes before a meal) diluted in some water.

Moringa

Moringa (Moringa oleifera) is a very special tree found in Africa and the Himalayas. It is often called "the wonder tree" or "Never Die", because of its numerous health benefits and its absolute sturdiness and resistance. As it turns out, Moringa has the exact same effects on our bodies as well. It builds our natural immunity and makes us healthier and stronger with enhanced ability to counteract diseases and harsh environment. Moringa's fruits, leaves and oil are full of vitamins, minerals, and nutrients, which makes it a real superfood. For example, Moringa contains 4 times more Potassium than bananas, 2 times more vitamin A than carrots, and 2 times more fiber than oat meal. It also supplies us with Calcium, Magnesium, Phosphorus, Copper, Iron, Sulfur, Vitamin B1, B2, B3, C, E, important amino acids such as Arginine, Histidine, Lysine, Tryptophan, Phenylalanine, Methionine, Threonine, Leucine, Isoleucine, and Valine.

Moringa lowers the blood pressure, stimulates the metabolism, supports the digestive tract, soothes the nervous system, boosts the immunity and detoxes the body. The plant is excellent for vegetarians/vegans for its essential amino acids. According to the traditional Indian medicine (Ayurveda), Moringa can prevent, counteract and heal us from more than 3000 health conditions and ailments. It also stimulates the digestion and fights anxiety and insomnia. It gently detoxifies the body and strengthens the immune system. The herb is even suitable for diabetics. Moringa, just like Zeloite, we talked about in book 1 of the series, is a powerful water purifier – it sterilizes it and eliminates the staphylococci and streptococci (often resistant to antibiotics). Moringa is an excellent nutrient for vegetarians/vegans, active athletes, and fastidious children.

You can add this superfood to your diet in various ways – add Moringa powder in your smoothie, juice, soup, desserts, or cook the plant directly.

Here are a couple of recipes you can try at home:

Vegan Soup with Moringa

Ingredients:
4 Tbsps. dices **carrots**
4 Tbsps. dices/grated **celery root**
1 small **onion**
2 cloves **garlic**
10 slices **dry tomatoes**
2 Tbsps. **dry Moringa powder**
2-3 Tbsps. **sunflower or olive oil** for cooking
Some **salt and pepper**

Directions:

Dice the onion and the garlic. Mix them with the carrots, celery, the oil, and some water in a pot. Stew the veggies until they become softer. Add 2 cups water and the dry tomatoes. Let the mixture simmer for half an hour on low heat. Then, blend the soup with a hand blender and add the moringa, the salt, and the pepper. Enjoy!

Healthy Muffins

Ingredients:
1 cup **wholegrain flour**
2 tsps. **baking soda**
2 tsps. **stevia**
3 Tbsps. **coconut butter**
1/2 cup **nut milk**
1 tsp. **allspice**
1 tsp. **nutmeg**
1 tsp. organic **vanilla extract**
1 Tbsp. **Moringa powder**
5-6 Tbsps. **cranberries**

Directions:

In a bowl mix the flour, baking soda, stevia, allspice, vanilla, and the moringa. In another pot, melt the coconut butter, mix it with the nut milk and stir well. Combine the dry and the liquid ingredients and blend them completely. Use a mixer if necessary. Add the cranberries and stir again. Pour the mixture in your molds, and fill them at about 2/3 of their capacity. Sprinkle some nutmeg powder on top and put them in the preheated oven. The temperature needs to be 180 Celsius (356 Fahrenheit). Bake for about 20-25 minutes and voila!

More Immune Boosting Tactics

"Health is a state of complete harmony of the body, mind and spirit. When one is free from physical disabilities and mental distractions, the gates of the soul open."

~B.K.S. Iyengar

Reflexology for stronger immunity

Reflexology is an alternative healing system based on the ancient Chinese holistic medicine. This traditional Eastern medicine is focused on the energy system of the human body. It is comprised of energy circuits called meridians. Each meridian has a certain end point. When the energy flow is disrupted (for example from an emotional trauma or illness), these end points are being punctured with special needles (acupuncture) or pressed (acupressure), thus healing the energy system and restoring its balance. Although it may sound a bit woo-woo for the logical mind, this healing system has been proven extremely effective time and time again.

While acupuncture can be conducted only by professionals, reflexology is much more simple and applicable for the common folk. It consists of simple massages on the feet, hands, and ears, stimulating the blood, lymph flow, and more importantly – the energy flow of the body.

The 6 points in the pinna

In reflexology, there are 6 main points in the auricle, which are known to stimulate the immunity. Fortunately, we do not need to know their exact spots. All we need to do is to gently massage both pinnae several times a day. Try to keep the movements from the top of the ear downward to the soft spot of the pinna. This massage will gently stimulate the blood flow and boost the natural immune response.

The fourth finger

Massages of the fourth finger (the ring finger) also have a wonderful stimulating effect. Reflexology experts say that 200 massaging strokes from the top to the base of the finger will be enough for prevention.

"A walk at the shore"

The feet are the most common used body parts for reflexology. They have numerous healing points we can use at our disposal. That is why walking barefoot is recommended even from the conventional medicine. But what if we do not have access to the beach or the weather is too cold? One option is to make a simple foot massage. Or another option is to emulate the walk on the beach at home. Here is how to do it. Take some decorative oval sea pebbles and place them in a laundry basin. Cover the stones with a solution of warm water, sea salt, and a few drops apple cider vinegar. Tread on the pebbles 3 times a day for at least 5 minutes. This procedure can be applied even for small children.

Essential oils for immunity

Reflexology massages can be even better and stronger with the help of essential oils. These floral extracts are extremely concentrated and should not be underestimated. I have talked a lot about their magical healing properties in

"Toxin-free Homemade Beauty Recipes" and in book 2 of the Detox and Immunity series ("Complete Body Cleansing: lymph detox, juicing cleanse, parasite flush, kidney purification, liver detox, and more") you can find how to use them for a nice gentle cleansing detox massage.

Here we will explore their magical properties to strengthen our system and build our immunity. The best essential oils for this purpose are:

- **Tea tree** – this oil is extremely powerful – it has soothing, regenerating, antiseptic, antifungal, antibacterial, anti-itching, and healing properties. It also works for lowering high temperature and as a bug repellent. It stimulates the immune system, and counteracts viral infections, flu, colds, tonsillitis, coughs, sinusitis, asthma, throat and gum infections, and mouth ulcers; prevents from plaque and formation of tartar, bad breath, etc. Tea tree oil has the power to regenerate the skin cells, shrink the pores (excellent for blackhead treatments), fight acne, infected wounds, herpes, warts; it soothes insect bites, burns, itching, sweaty feet, cystitis, vaginal discharge and inflammations. It also tones the heart, stimulates the blood circulation, and can be used in addition to varicose veins treatments.

  Consult with a physician before using this oil if you have hormone sensitive conditions, if you are pregnant or breastfeeding.

  Preparation of the massage oil: mix 3 Tbsps. (50 ml) of a carrier oil of choice (almond, avocado, apricot, grape seed, etc.) with 25 drops Tea tree essential oil. Stir well and gently massage the body as you pay extra attention to the lymph nodes.

- **Eucalyptus** – this oil is antibacterial, regenerating, invigorating, toning, analgesic, antiseptic, stimulating, refreshing, diuretic, and antiviral. It helps us relieve and prevent from colds, a runny nose, sore throat, all kinds of respiratory problems, lowers the body temperature, reduces the fever, infections, boosts the metabolism, and helps with strengthening our immune system. It could soothe severe headaches and stimulate our ability to concentrate. Eucalyptus oil is suitable for treating skin infections, herpes, cuts and burns. It is extremely valuable for the joints and muscles - reduces the tension and helps people with arthritis and rheumatism. It is an excellent disinfectant.

  The preparation of the massage oil is the same as the previous one – 25 drops essential oil with 3 Tbsps. carrier oil. Concentrate on the chest area to maximize its benefits.

- **Cinnamon** – this is a wonderful refreshing, exciting, energizing, antidepressant, antiseptic, detoxing, antispasmodic, carminative, styptic, blood circulation boosting, disinfecting, warming, and deodorizing essential oil. It stimulates the immune system, prevents from colds, coughs, and respiratory inflammations. Soothes the dizziness and nausea. The oil counteracts bad breath, stimulates the blood circulation and the cells' nutrition (excellent for mature skin), speeds the metabolism, and fights cellulite.

The preparation of the massage oil is the same as the previous one.

- **Clove** – the essential oil has excellent toning, antiseptic, antibacterial, analgesic, warming, immune boosting, carminative, anti-oxidative, digestion stimulating, aphrodisiac, and bug repelling properties. Clove oil adjusts the level of unsaturated fatty acids in our bodies and prevents from their fast aging and deterioration. It soothes muscle tension and injuries, rheumatism, and arthritis. It can be used to treat skin wounds and ulcers, and bites from insects. Clove essential oil is also effective for different kinds of digestive disorders, bloating, and flatulence; against oral infections, gingivitis, periodontitis, bad breath. flu, cough, tonsillitis, fever, and many more.

  Preparation of the massage oil: mix 3 Tbsps. (50 ml) of a carrier oil of choice (almond, avocado, apricot, jojoba, etc.) with 10-15 drops Clove essential oil.

The extracts from ***Anise, Lemon (or Lime), Oregano, Rosemary, White camphor, Balsam fir (Abies balsamea), Ginger, Citronella, Ravensara (Ravensara aromatica), Immortelle (Helichrysum italicum)***, can also do wonders for the immune system.

Immune Boosting Recipes

"Let food be thy medicine and medicine be thy food"
~Hippocrates

In this chapter you will find lots of recipes, natural remedies, strengthening potions, and healing mixtures that will boost your immunity and prevent from various disease developments.

Vitaminful mixture

Ingredients:
1.5 cup **raisins**
1 cup **walnuts**
1/2 cup **almonds**
2 **lemons**
1/2 cup **raw honey**

Directions:

Soak the nuts in clean water and let them sit overnight. The next day, strain them and wash them thoroughly. Next, remove the skin of the lemons and squeeze their juice in a cup. Place the nuts, lemon zest, the lemon juice, and the honey in a mincer or a chopper until you get a homogenous mixture. Place the substance in a glass jar with a lid. Put the jar in a dark and cool place for 2 days and the immune boosting recipe is ready.

Take 1 Tbsp. 3 times a day 1 hour before a meal. For small children the dosage is 1-2 tsps.

Immune boosting recipe with bran

Ingredients:
1 Tbsp. **wheat or rye bran**
1 cup **pure water**
1 Tbsp. dry **Calendula blossom**
1 tsp. **raw honey**

Directions:

Boil the bran in the water for 30-40 minutes. Next, add the Calendula blossom and let the mixture simmer for 5 more minutes. Next, take it off the heat, let it cool off and strain with a strainer or cheesecloth. Add the honey. Divide the drink in 2-3 parts and drink those 30 minutes before each meal.

Prepare a fresh batch each day.

Immune boosting recipe with cranberries

Ingredients:
1 kilo (4 cups) **fresh cranberries**
2 **lemons**
1 cup **raw organic honey**

Directions:

Cut the lemons in large pieces and remove the seeds. Next, place them in a mincer or kitchen chopper. Add the cranberries and mince them well. Add the honey and stir until you have a nice homogenous mixture. Place the remedy in a glass jar.

Take 1-2 Tbsps. 2-3 times a day before a meal. You can mix it with some healing tea (for example field horsetail infusion).

Immune boosting and detoxing recipe from Marva Oganyan

Ingredients:
1 kilo (4 cups) **fresh young Stinging nettle**
2 **lemons**
2 **apples**
Some **raw honey** according to your taste
Stinging nettle tea

Directions:

It is important for the Stinging nettle to be fresh and young – gathered in the spring when the leaves are still small. Wash the nettle leaves gently or soak them in some pure water to remove any dust or dirt. Cut the lemons in pieces and remove the seeds. Cut the apples in large chunks as well. It will be easier for them to be minced. Place the green leaves, the apples and lemons in a blender, add some of the Stinging nettle tea and puree them until the mixture becomes smooth. Add more tea if you need to in order to reach a nice smoothie consistency. Add the honey and stir well again. Store in a large glass jar in the fridge.

Take 1 cup of the smoothie 2 times a day (for example in the morning and in the evening) before a meal.

Strong Immunity with a simple Fig Syrup

Ingredients:
100 grams (1/2 cup) **fresh or dried figs**
2 cups **pure water**

Directions:

Mince the figs and pour the water onto them. Put the mixture on the stove and let it simmer for about 15 minutes on low heat. Next, take the infusion off the heat and put a lid on the container and steep the figs for 2 hours.

Take 100 ml (6 Tbsps.) of the syrup 3 times a day before a meal. Do not add any sugar, honey or sweeteners.

This natural remedy will help the work of the gastrointestinal tract; boost your vitality and productivity. For best results try to apply this remedy for at least 4 days.

Green Walnuts Syrup

Ingredients:
10 **"young" green walnuts**
2 **clove buds**
1 kilo (4 cups) **raw organic honey**
1 liter (4 cups) **pure water**

Directions:

You need young green walnuts which are still small with soft shells. Dice the walnuts in small pieces, as small as possible. Be careful, though, they will stain your hands and clothes. So, put on rubber gloves and an apron.

Next, place the walnuts in a metal pot and pour the water in it. Put the pot on the stove and let the mixture simmer for about 10 minutes. Add the clove buds and put the pot off the heat. Let the mixture cool off to body temperature and add the honey. Stir well until the honey is fully melted and dissolved. Pour the syrup in glass bottles and seal them tight. Store in a dark and cool place.

Take 1 tsp. 3 times a day after a meal.

This syrup can successfully boost your natural immunity and fight chronic fatigue and gastrointestinal issues.

Very important notice: this remedy contains large amounts of Iodine. Anyone who has any type of problems with the thyroid should be very careful. If you have hypothyroidism, this recipe may even help you, but consult with your physician first! This rule applies for those who have relatives, especially parents or grandparents with thyroid diseases. In that case, it is advisable for you to check your gland and consult with your doctor about taking this walnut remedy.

Wheat Grass Smoothie

Ingredients:
1-2 **bananas**
A fistful of **spinach**
1 tsp. **wheat grass powder**
2 **dates**
A pinch of **cinnamon**

Directions:

Place all ingredients in a blender and mix until you reach a nice homogenous smooth consistency.

Wheat grass is extremely beneficial for our health and immunity. It contains lots of vitamins, minerals, enzymes and essential amino acids. It has the power to heal various gastrointestinal issues and fight fatigue, exhaustion and low immunity.

Boost Your Immunity with Aloe Vera

Ingredients:
1 Tbsp. **Aloe Vera gel**
1 Tbsp. **raw organic honey**
The quantities are for one dose.

Directions:

Mix the Aloe and honey well and take 30 minutes before a meal. Take this healthy mixture 3 times a day for 10 consecutive days. Next, take a 10-day break and repeat the procedure.

If you have an Aloe Plant at home (Aloe Barbadensis Miller), you can use its fresh gel straight from its leaves.

Immunity and Eyesight Boosting Smoothie

Ingredients:

100-150 ml (~1/2 cup) **fresh tangerine juice**
3 **carrots**
1/2 **mango**

Directions:

Wash the carrots and the mango thoroughly and peel them. Cut them in large pieces and place them in the blender. Add the tangerine juice and mince them well. When you reach a nice smooth consistency, the smoothie is ready!

This drink is excellent for immune boosting, strengthening the eyesight and prevention from various diseases.

Fruit Smoothie

Ingredients:
1/2 cup **strawberries**
1/2 cup **pineapple**
1 ripe **banana**

Directions:
Peel the banana and cut in pieces along with the pineapple. Place all ingredients in a blender and mix. If you need to, you can add some pure water for easier blending. Enjoy!

Nutty Good Immune Mix 1

Ingredients:
1 kilo (4 cups) **raw organic honey**
500 ml (2 cups) **lemon juice**, freshly squeezed
350 grams (1 1/2 cup) **sesame tahini**
250 grams (1 cup) **raw hazelnuts**
250 grams (1 cup) **raw almonds**
250 grams (1 cup) **raw walnuts**
250 grams (1 cup) **raw sesame seeds**
30 ml (2 Tbsps.) **propolis tincture**
10 grams (2 tsps.) **cinnamon powder** (or grated nutmeg)

Directions:

Grind the nuts and sesame seeds in a mincer or kitchen chopper. Next, place the honey in a large glass jar with a lid. Add the sesame tahini and the lemon juice and stir well until everything becomes fully homogenous. Add all other remaining ingredients and stir well again. After everything is fully blended, seal the jar tight and place it in a dark and cool place.

Take 1 tsp. of the mixture 4 times a day – before breakfast, lunch, dinner, and before bed.

Nutty Good Immune Mix 2

Ingredients:

500 grams (2 cups) **raw organic honey**
1 lemon
50 grams (1.7 oz.) **raw hazelnuts**
50 grams (1.7 oz.) **raw almonds**
50 grams (1.7 oz.) **raw walnuts**
50 grams (1.7 oz.) **raisins**
50 grams (1.7 oz.) **grated horseradish**

Directions:

Grind all the nuts and the raisins. Squeeze the juice from the lemon. Place the honey in a large glass jar with a tight lid. Add all other ingredients and stir well. Seal the jar and store it in the fridge.

Take 1 Tbsp. twice a day (morning and evening) an hour after a meal.

When the remedy is over, make another batch and repeat the healing course. This natural immune booster is excellent for the Fall in preparation for the cold months, and during winter itself for flu prevention.

Lemon Cream

Ingredients:
2 **lemons**
200 grams (7 oz.) **brown or coconut sugar**
60 grams (4 Tbsps.) **unsalted bio butter**
3 **eggs**

Directions:

Divide the sugar in two halves. Take one half and grind it until you reach a powder consistency. A food processor, coffee grinder, or a powerful blender work well. Peel the lemons and grate their zest and squeeze the juice out of them. Next, mix the two types of sugar, the butter, the grated lemon zests, and the lemon juice. In another container stir the eggs and add them to the sugary mixture. Stir it well until it is fully blended. Place the pot in a double boiler on low heat and continue stirring until the sugar melts completely. It should take about 10 minutes. Remember not to let the mixture boil for it will burn the ingredients. Pour the cream (while it is still hot) in small glass jars with screw lids. Place the jars upside down and let them cool off. The hot air will create vacuum that will preserve the cream for a longer period. Place the jars in a dark and cool place or in the fridge for not longer than 2-3 months.

Take 1 tbsp. of the cream first thing in the morning. This recipe is suitable even for kids, and it will be a fun and delicious way to keep their immunity strong and prevent them from colds and the flu.

Weight-loss and Immunity Shake

Ingredients:
1/2 **pineapple**
1 **banana**
400 ml (1 1/2 cup) **probiotic yogurt**
2 **oranges**

Directions:
Peel the fruits and cut them in large pieces. Place them in a blender or a food processor, and add the yogurt. Mince everything well until it is fully blended and homogenous. This batch can be stored in the fridge (in the summer) and taken throughout the day.

Persimmon Shake

Ingredients:
100-200 ml (1/2 cup) **probiotic yogurt**
4 **oranges**
2 **persimmons**
1 tsp. **organic raw honey**
A few **fresh Mint leaves** (optional)

Directions:

Wash the fruits thoroughly and squeeze the juice from the oranges. Peel the persimmons and cut them in large pieces. Put them in a blender and add the yogurt and the orange juice. Mix the ingredients well until they form a homogenous mass. Pour in a glass container and add the honey. Stir until the honey melts completely. Decorate the drink with the Mint leaves. Drink this potion immediately after preparation.

The Ultimate Health Recipe

Ingredients:

100 grams (~1/2 cup) **flax seeds**
100 grams (~1/2 cup) **raw sesame seeds**
100 grams (~1/2 cup) **raw sunflower seeds** (peeled)
Bulgarian or Greek **yogurt**
Flax seed oil (optional)
Apple pectin powder (optional)
Honey (optional)
Bee pollen (optional)

Directions:

Mix the seeds and grind them. Store the “flour” in a sealable glass jar. In the evening take 1 Tbsp. of the seed powder and mix it with 2 Tbsps. yogurt. Let the mixture sit overnight and eat it in the morning on an empty stomach. If you like to boost this recipe, you can add 1 Tbsp. flax seed oil, 1 tsp. apple pectin powder, 1 tsp. honey, and 1/2 tsp. bee pollen. Add more yogurt if needed.

Note: if you add the bee pollen, you need to soak it in the yogurt overnight with the seeds.

Powerful Immunity Boosting Toner

Ingredients:

700 ml (2 1/2 cups) natural **apple cider vinegar**
1/4 cup minced **onions**
1/4 cup minced **garlic**
2 **fresh peppers**, diced
1/4 cup grated **ginger root**
2 Tbsps. **grated horseradish**
2 Tbsps. **turmeric**

Directions:

Take a large glass jar with a screw lid. Place all vegetables inside. The jar needs to be big enough so that they take 2/3 of its capacity. Pour the apple cider vinegar to fully submerse them and fill the jar to the top. Put the jar in a dry and well ventilated place and shake it twice a day for at least 2 weeks. Next, strain the mixture with cheesecloth and pour the liquid in a tightly sealed bottle or a jar. Store the toner in a cool and dark place.

Take 1 Tbsp. a day after a meal. You can eat a citrus fruit afterwards to soothe your taste buds from the spicy toner. Do not dilute it in water for it will lower its potency.

Important: this toner may not be suitable for people with sensitive stomachs or any other gastrointestinal issues. Consult with a physician in such cases. Do not take this liquid on an empty stomach!

This recipe is extremely powerful and potent! It is one of the strongest natural antibiotics, which does not harm the beneficial gut flora. On the contrary, the acidity from the apple cider vinegar will promote its growth and health. It has anti-viral and anti-fungal properties. This acid infusion saved countless lives in the past preventing and healing from various epidemics. It stimulates the blood and lymph flow and counteracts even the most stubborn health issues, like the Candida infections.

Weight-loss Detoxifier

Ingredients:
1/2 tsp. **cayenne pepper powder**
1 lemon
1 cup **pure water**
A little **raw honey** (optional)

Directions:

Squeeze the juice from the lemon and mix it with the cayenne pepper. Add the water and stir well. If the taste is too strong and sour for you, you can add some honey to the mix.

Take this potion first thing in the morning on an empty stomach for one week.

Important: this drink may not be suitable for people with sensitive stomachs or any other gastrointestinal issues.

Cayenne peppers are famous for their healing and boosting properties. They stimulate the blood flow and promote natural cleansing and weight-loss.

Purslane Pickles

Ingredients:

250 ml (1 cup) raw organic **apple cider vinegar**

250 grams (1 cup) **fresh purslane** (Portulaca oleracea)

10 grains **black pepper**

3 cloves **garlic**

Directions:

Try to find the purest purslane you can find and wash it thoroughly. Place it in a jar and add the garlic and pepper seeds. Pour the apple cider vinegar to submerse the plants and seal it with the lid. Put the jar in the fridge for about 2 weeks and the pickles are ready!

Purslane is a wonderful natural supplement to any healthy diet plan. It is considered a weed, but it holds much more power than we suspect. It can be called a super food that costs you nothing – it is growing almost everywhere. You can even add this valuable plant in your own outside or inside garden.

And the good news is, purslane does not need much care and fertilizing.

Consider adding this herb in your diet because of its numerous beneficial nutrients – Omega-3 Fatty acids, vitamins (B1, B2, B3), minerals (Copper, Phosphorus), and folic acid. You can successfully add this leafy plant in your green smoothies and healthy meals.

Healthy Chocolate Candy

Ingredients:
1 1/4 cup **coconut butter**
1/4 cup **honey**
1/2 tsp. **liquid Mint extract**
90-100 grams (1/2 cup) **bio dark chocolate** (without sugar or artificial sweeteners)

Directions:

Take 1 cup of the coconut butter, the honey and the Mint extract and mix them well in a pot. From this dough form small balls. Place the coconut balls in a tray covered with oiled paper. Put the tray in the fridge for 10-15 minutes. In the meantime, melt the chocolate in a double boiler on low temperature. Add the remaining coconut butter. Stir well the ingredients and take them off the heat. Wait for the liquid to cool off for a couple of minutes. Take the coconut balls out of the fridge. Dip each ball in the chocolate mass and place it back on the oiled paper. After all candies are covered, put the tray back in the fridge for the chocolate to harden completely. And voila!

The honey will stimulate the immunity in a gentle way. The coconut butter will supply essential fats and boost the metabolism. While the Mint will soothe any respiratory problem. And let's not forget all the wonderful benefits of the natural dark chocolate – it protects our immunity, the cardiovascular system, stimulates the brain, etc.

Healthy Chocolate Bars (Yay!)

Ingredients:
3/4 cup **cocoa butter**
6 Tbsps. **cocoa**
2 Tbsps. Grade B **maple syrup**
2 tsps. **vanilla**
A pinch of **Himalayan salt**

Directions:

Put the cocoa butter in a double boiler and melt it. Remember not to let the water boil and burn the butter. Add all other ingredients and stir well. After the mixture is well blended, pour it in silicon forms with the desired shape. Put the forms in the fridge until the chocolate hardens. Next, remove the bars from the forms and store them in a glass container with a tight lid in the fridge. But I am sure they won't survive for long.

This cocoa deliciousness will strengthen the cardiovascular system, boost the natural immunity, and lower the cholesterol and blood sugar levels. It contains Magnesium, which supports the nervous system, the bones, joints and the teeth. And also Copper – regulates the metabolism and prevents from premature grey hair.

Green Smoothie for Immunity

Ingredients:
1 cup fresh **apple juice**
2 cups minced **kale**
2 cups **strawberries**
Some **Aloe Vera gel**

Directions:

If you have an Aloe Barbadensis Miller plant at home, you can take one big leaf and extract its gel. If not, take some bio Aloe Vera gel from the health stores and add it to this smoothie mix. The optimum daily amounts are 60-90 ml. (2-3 oz.).

Place all ingredients in a blender and mix until they blend completely. Take the smoothie immediately.

This healthy drink will supply you with a plethora of vitamins, minerals, and enzymes! It will boost your immunity in no time!

Hemp Milk Toner

Ingredients:
1 mango
1 Tbsp. **bee pollen**
1/2 tsp. **turmeric powder**
1/2 tsp. **coconut butter**
1/2 cup **hemp milk**

Directions:

Peel the mango and extract the flesh of the fruit. Cut it in large pieces and put it in the blender. Add all the other ingredients and blend them well until you reach a nice consistency. Drink immediately.

As you can see, this recipe is full of beneficial ingredients that will boost your natural immunity and fight chronic fatigue and sluggishness.

Healthy Jelly Beans

Ingredients:
2 Tbsps. **pure water**
2 Tbsps. high quality **gelatin**
2 Tbsps. fresh **lemon juice**
2 Tbsps. **raw honey**

Directions:

Mix the water and the gelatin in a double boiler on low heat. Remember not to let the water boil or simmer. Add the lemon juice and the honey. Stir until the honey melts completely and the consistency is fully homogenous. Pour the liquid in proper silicon forms and place them in the fridge for several hours.

If you and your kids like this recipe, you can increase the quantities and use various fun forms. After the candies are ready, put them in a glass jar with tight lid and store them in the fridge.

Beside the lemons and honey, which have proven health benefits, gelatin is also a substance that is extremely valuable for us. It strengthens the ligaments, the hair, nails, and skin. It improves our appearance with its anti-age properties, and keeps us flexible and agile.

Dandelion Syrup

Ingredients:

2 cups **strawberries**
1 cup **bio balsamic vinegar**
1 cup **apple cider vinegar**
1/2 cup **Dandelion roots**
1/2 cup **raw honey**
2 Tbsps. grated **ginger root**

Directions:

Wash the strawberries and cut them in pieces. Put them in a pot and mash them with a wooden spoon or a masher. Dice the Dandelion roots and add them to the strawberries. In another container mix the vinegars and the honey. Stir until the honey is completely melted. Add the sweet liquid to the strawberry mix. Stir all ingredients well. Place the mixture in a glass jar with a lid. The lid should not be metal or have any metal parts. The vinegar might damage them and infiltrate the mixture. Place the jar in the fridge for a week. Next, strain the infusion and put it in a glass bottle with a tight lid. Store in a cool and dry place not more than 6 months.

Take 1-2 Tbsps. from the syrup diluted in some water daily.

Elderberry Potion

Ingredients:

3/4 cup **dry Elderberry fruits**
3 cups **pure water**
1 cup **raw honey**
1 tsp. **grated ginger root**
1 **cinnamon stick**
4 **clove buds**

Directions:

Place the elderberries, the water, ginger, cinnamon, and the clove buds in a pot. Place it on the stove and heat it until it starts to boil. Let it simmer for about 30 minutes. Next, take it off the heat and let it cool off a little bit. Strain the mixture with cheesecloth. After the infusion's temperature drops down to body temperature, add the honey. Stir well until the honey melts (preferably with a wooden utensil). Pour the syrup in a bottle with a tight lid. Store in a dark and cool place.

Take 1 Tbsp. daily. You can add this magical immune boosting potion to your smoothies or shakes.

This recipe is full of beneficial nutrients like antioxidants, Calcium, Phosphorus, Potassium, Vitamin C, etc. It is absolutely perfect for the winter season, preventing from the flu and soothing all kinds of respiratory issues.

Celtic Immune Boosting Tea Blend

Ingredients:
1 Tbsp. **dry Rosehips**
1 Tbsp. **dry raspberries**
1 Tbsp. **Melissa**
1 Tbsp. **Mint**
1 Tbsp. **Thyme**
1 Tbsp. **Echinacea**
400 ml (2 cups) **pure water**

Directions:

Put the water in a metal pot and bring it to boil. Add the herbs and fruits and let them simmer for 10 minutes. Strain the infusion and store it in a glass jar or bottle in the fridge.

Take 100 ml (1/2 cup) of this tea daily on empty stomach. You can divide the quantity in 2 parts and take 50 ml before breakfast and before bed.

This tea blend not only will boost your immunity naturally, but will also calm and strengthen your nervous system as well.

Immune Boosting Tea Blend 2

Ingredients:
1 Tbsp. **Salvia**
1 Tbsp. **Melilot**
1 Tbsp. **Primrose**
1 Tbsp. **Sarsaparilla**
1 Tbsp. **Calendula**
1 Tbsp. **Field Horsetail**
1 Tbsp. **Common Agrimony**

Directions:

Mix all herbs in a glass container with a tight lid. Take 2 Tbsps. of the blend and steep them in 600 ml (~ 2 cups) boiling water. Let the infusion cool off. Take 100 ml (1/2 cup) of the tea 3 times a day half an hour before a meal.

Cardiovascular Fruit Smoothie

Ingredients:
15 **bilberries (blueberries)**
30 **grapes**
10 **strawberries**
8 **cranberries**
1/2 **apple**
5 **aronia fruits or black currant**
1 **peach or a kiwi**

Directions:

Wash the fruits and place them in a blender. Mince them until the mixture is homogenous. Divide the smoothie in 2-3 parts and take each one before a meal. Make a new batch each day.

This recipe is devised by French scientists. They came to the conclusion that these ingredients have the power to activate our natural immune response, stimulate the blood circulation, preventing from heart diseases. This smoothie can be used for prevention, and as a recovery remedy.

Blueberry wine

Ingredients:

1 liter (4 cups) **bio red wine** (aronia wine is a perfect option)
1/2 liter (2 cups) **brandy**
1/2 kilo (2 cups) **blueberries**
1/2 kilo (2 cups) **juniper berries**
3 Tbsps. **brown or coconut sugar**
3 Tbsps. **raw honey**

Directions:

Wash the fruits carefully and place them in a large glass jar. Pour the wine in the container and seal it. Let the fruits ferment at room temperature for 48 hours. Next, add the brandy, sugar and honey. Stir the mixture until the honey and the sugar are completely dissolved. Seal the jar again and let it sit for one more week. The wine is ready.

Take 4 Tbsps. of the mixture 2 times a day for 3 days. Try to add a couple of fruits to each dosage. Pause for 2 days and repeat the course. You can follow this schedule until you finish the liquor.

This recipe may not be suitable when driving or operating machinery. Consult with your physician first.

Siberian Immune Remedy

Ingredients:
2/3 cup **pine needles**
2/3 cup **fir needles**
2/3 cup **cedar needles**
1 Tbsp. **oregano**
A fistful of **Rosehip fruits**
1 tsp. minced **raspberry leaves**
1 liter (4 cups) **pure water**

Directions:

Place all plants in a pot with a lid. Bring the water to the boiling point and pour it onto all ingredients. Put the lid on and let them steep for 3-4 hours. Next, strain the mixture, and the healing tea is ready.

Take 150 ml (1/2 cup) 2 times a day on an empty stomach. You can add some honey or cranberries to improve its taste.

Pumpkin Honey

Ingredients:
1 fully **ripe orange pumpkin**
Honey, brown sugar, or coconut sugar

Directions:

Cut the top of the pumpkin, but do not throw it away – we will need it as a lid later on. Scoop out all seeds and fiber. Next, fill the pumpkin with the honey or sugar. Put the "lid" on and place the filled pumpkin in a pot or a big plate and store it in a cool and dry place. The honey will be ready when the pumpkin starts to become soft. It means the honey/sugar has soaked and drained enough of the healthy pumpkin juice. When the sweet nectar is fully dissolved, scoop it out and store it in a glass container with a tight lid in the fridge. If the remaining pumpkin pulp is in a good shape, you can bake it in the oven as a nice healthy dessert.

Take 2-3 Tbsps. from the pumpkin honey daily. You can also add it in desserts, smoothies and teas. If you used the honey for this recipe, remember not to heat it over the body temperature.

Pumpkins are one of the best healthy products during the Fall. They are full of vitamins and Carotene, helping us boost our immunity before the winter and strengthening our eyesight. Its juice has a nice gentle diuretic effect, and it is perfect for people with constipation. It prevents from various diseases.

Note: do not throw away the pumpkin seeds! You can use them in the Immune Boosting Vitamin

Bomb (see below) or as a natural anti-parasite remedy (see book 2 "Complete Body Cleansing" of the series).

Healing Pine Elixir

Ingredients:
100 **pine buds** (0.4-0.7 inches) or **young green pine cones** (0.7-1.2 inch)
1 kilo (4 cups) **coconut sugar** or Grade B **maple syrup**
1 tsp. **citric acid powder**
2 liters (8 cups) **pure water**

Directions:

Take the pine buds (or pine cones) and place them in a metal pot. Pour the water in and heat it. Let the infusion simmer until half of the water evaporates. (If you use pine buds, you can mash them at his point.) Next, strain the mixture and put the pine infused water back on the stove. Add the sugar (or maple syrup) and heat it until it thickens. The color of the elixir should become dark brown. Now add the citric acid, stir well and take off the heat. Pour in glass jars and seal them.

This recipe could be modified for different kinds of buds and cones – for example fir or spruce.

Dragon Cider for Bulletproof Immunity

Ingredients:

1/2 cup grated **horseradish**
1/2 cup grated **ginger root**
1 **onion**, diced
10 **garlic cloves**, mashed
4-5 cm (1.5-2 inch) **turmeric root**, grated
1 **lemon**
Spices according to your preferences – **Rosemary, Cayenne pepper, Cinnamon**
Raw organic **apple cider vinegar**
Raw honey

Directions:

Cut the lemon in pieces and put it in a large glass jar. Add all other ingredients. Pour the apple cider vinegar until you fill the jar completely. Wrap the top of the jar with a tissue. Do not use a metal cap/lid. Store the jar in a dark and cool place for a month. Shake the mixture once in a while. Next, after the one month period, strain the infusion with cheesecloth and add some honey to sweeten its taste. Pour it in a glass bottle (preferably with a cork cap).

For prevention: take 1 Tbsp. of the Dragon cider daily.

In cases of flu/colds: take 1 Tbsp. 3 times a day in addition to your therapy. Consult with your physician first!

Yummy Tahini Balls

Ingredients:

1 part **sesame tahini** or **ground sesame seeds**

1 part **raw honey**

Whole **sesame seeds**

Directions:

Mix the tahini and the honey until you reach a dough-like consistency. Form round balls and cover them with the sesame seeds. Next, place them in a glass container with a lid and put them in the fridge for them to keep their form.

Take 1-2 balls on an empty stomach.

These delicious candies will help you tremendously in multiple ways. They will strengthen the natural immunity, supply important nutrients, prevent from osteoporosis, lower the cholesterol levels, fight chronic fatigue, and heal gastritis and ulcers.

Immune Boosting Vitamin Bomb

Ingredients:

1/2 cup **raisins**

A fistful of **raw pumpkin seeds**

1 cup **raw walnuts**

1/2 cup **raw almonds**

2 **lemons**

1/4 cup **dry plums**

1/4 cup **dry apricots**

150 grams (1/2 cup) **raw honey**

Directions:

Mince the dry plums and apricots. Squeeze the juice from the lemons (do not throw away the zest). Mix the plums, apricots, lemon juice and the honey. Stir until the honey is fully melted. Grind the nuts, pumpkin seeds, and the raisins. Grate the lemon peel, and mix everything in a large glass jar. Seal the jar and place it in a dark, dry, and cool place for 2 days. The remedy is ready – store it in the fridge.

For adults: take 1-2 Tbsps. 2-3 times a day.

For small kids: 1-2 tsps. 2-3 times a day. Consult with a pediatrician first!

Summer Refreshing Cranberreade

Ingredients:

1/2 liter (3 cups) **water**
100 ml (1/2 cup) **lemon juice**
100 grams (1/2 cup) **coconut sugar**
60 ml (2 oz.) **cranberry juice**

Directions:

Mix all ingredients in a glass pitcher and stir until the sugar is completely dissolved. Serve immediately or let it cool in the fridge.

Cardiovascular and Immunity Mix

Ingredients:

3 **lemons**
200 grams (~1 cup) **dry plums**
200 grams (~1 cup) **raisins**
200 grams (~1 cup) **dry apricots**
200 grams (~1 cup) **raw walnuts**
100 grams (1/2 cup) **Hawthorn fruits**
100 grams (1/2 cup) **Rosehip fruits**
250 grams (~1 cup) **raw honey**

Directions:

Wash the lemons thoroughly and cut them in large pieces. Remove the seeds and place them in a food processor or a mincer (with the zest). Add the plums, raisins, apricots, walnuts, hawthorn and rosehip fruits. After everything is minced well, put in a glass container with a lid. Add the honey and stir well.

Take 1 Tbsp. daily on an empty stomach.

This mixture is perfect for strengthening the heart and boosting the natural defense system. It can be used as a preventive tool or as a remedy for faster recovery from various diseases. It contains lots of Potassium – essential for our health, and the nutrients in Rosehips and Hawthorn sooth the nervous system as well.

Delicious Protein Immunity Bars

Ingredients:
1 cup **dates**
1 cup **pineapple**
1 1/2 cup **desiccated coconut**
2 cups **raw cashew**
2 Tbsps. **vanilla**
8 tsps. **turmeric**

Directions:
Remove the kernels of the dates. Place all ingredients in a food processor, except 1/2 cup of the desiccated coconut. Blend everything until its homogenous. Spread the “dough” and press it with a rolling pin. Cut it in the desired forms and dip the bars in the remaining desiccated coconut. Place all protein bars in the fridge for them to harden.

Detox Protein Bars

Ingredients:
1 cup **desiccated coconut**
1/2 cup **raw sesame seeds**
3 **bananas**
2 Tbsps. **coconut butter**
1 Tbsp. **spirulina powder**
1 Tbsp. **vanilla**
1/4 tsp. **Himalayan salt**

Directions:

Peel the bananas and cut them in large pieces. Put them in a food processor and add the spirulina, coconut butter, the salt and the vanilla. Mix everything well until it is homogenous. Next, place the mixture in a pot and add the sesame seeds and the desiccated coconut. Stir well. Put the "dough" in a large tray and spread it evenly. Cut it in squares and let the bars dry in a well-ventilated place. Or you can dry them in a dehydrator.

PomeGRANADE Chocolate Bars

Ingredients:

250 grams (~1 cup) **bio dark chocolate**
1 cup **pomegranate seeds**
1 Tbsp. grated **ginger root**
1/4 tsp. ground **Himalayan salt**

Directions:

Place the chocolate in a double boiler to melt. Remember not to let the water boil or it will burn the ingredients. Add 1/2 cup of the pomegranate seeds, the salt, and the ginger. Stir well until the mix is homogenous. Take a tray and cover it with oiled baking paper. Pour the chocolate mixture on top of it and spread it with a spoon. Sprinkle the remaining pomegranate seeds over and press them gently in order for them to stick. Place the tray in the fridge for about 30 minutes for the chocolate to harden. Next, cut or chip the chocolate bars and consume!

Bon Appetite!

Energy Chocolate Bars

Ingredients:
1/2 cup **cocoa powder**
1/2 cup **coconut butter**
1/2 cup **seeds/nuts mixture** (put whatever you have and like – raisins, raspberries, desiccated coconut, pumpkin seeds, sesame seeds, etc.)
1/4 cup ground **pistachios**
1/4 cup Grade B **maple syrup**

Directions:

Place the coconut butter in a double boiler and melt it (the stove must be on very low heat). Add the maple syrup and the cocoa powder. Take out a tray and cover it with backing paper (oiled). Spread the mixture on top of it. Sprinkle the seeds/nuts mix and place the tray in the fridge for a couple of hours. Next, cut the mixture in squares and enjoy!

Oatmeal Candy

Ingredients:
1 cup **dry cranberries**
1 cup **oatmeal**
1/2 cup **almond butter**
1/4 cup **raw honey**
1/2 cup **crushed raw almonds**
1/2 cup **crushed pistachios**
1 Tbsp. **ground flax seeds**

Directions:

Place all ingredients in a bowl and mix them well with a wooden utensil. Put the bowl in the fridge so that the "dough" will harden. Next, take it out and start forming balls (or any other shapes you like). Place the candy in a tray and place it back in the fridge for several more minutes. Then you can serve the healthy desserts or place them in a glass jar and store it in the fridge

Healing detox and immunity recipes

"To keep the body in good health is a duty...
otherwise we shall not be able to keep our mind strong and clear."
~Buddha

In this chapter we will explore specific detox regimens and recipes which hold enormous power – the power to heal our bodies and restore our wellbeing. These are recipes tried and tested by many people around the world who were desperate to return to health and happiness. Most of these healing practices deal with difficult, sometimes even impossible cases of cancer, but they could work for almost all kinds of diseases and discomforts. What is their secret? Why these simple natural regimens can do what traditional medicine sometimes fails to achieve? The answer is simple and obvious – by deeply cleansing our bodies and supplying it with essential nutrients we activate our own immune system. And this absolutely perfect defense mechanism does what it was programmed to do – to restore, repair, heal, and evacuate the biological waste and pathogenic microorganisms.

But why our highly advanced medical industry in some cases cannot substitute the natural approach? My point of view is simple, and you are not obliged to agree with it. Modern medicine has become a pharmaceutical dealer, prescribing pills we do not necessarily need. For example, the alarming frequent usage of antibiotics - this leads to bacteria becoming more resistant and mutating into super bacteria. In her report researching the topic of bacteria's antibiotic resistance, Professor Dame Sally Davies warns us (and the medical industry): *"Antimicrobial resistance poses a catastrophic threat. If we don't act now, any one of us could go into hospital in 20 years for minor surgery and die because of an ordinary infection that can't be treated by antibiotics. And routine operations like hip replacements or organ transplants could be deadly because of the risk of infection."*

In addition to this statement I just want to remind that every drug we take, even just a small Aspirin, consists of complex chemical compounds. And most of them are not absorbed fully by our digestive tract. So, what happens to them? They get stuck in the liver, loading our workaholic body filter with even more work to do. Sadly, this applies even for many artificial food additives, "dead" vitamins, and minerals, unrecognizable by our system.

Having said that, I need to clarify I am not against traditional medicine! The natural and conventional approaches should not be opposed to each other. They need to work together for the sake of humanity. That is why I always advise people to consult with their physician before embarking on a new alternative healing program, or before making big changes in their diet and lifestyle. Modern medicine definitely has its part in improving our health. It does an excellent job of detecting unsymptomatic conditions in their initial stages, or performing state of the art procedures and operations only professionals can do, and so on. The key is in the balance.

Let's end this discussion for now, and jump into what you are here to do – learn how to naturally detox and heal your body. And below you can find recipes which helped lots of people achieve the exact same goal, and most importantly – that saved their lives!

Cancer healing cleansing methods

Sadly, due to our busy lifestyles full of junk foods and stress, cancer has become a real plague among us. Even though we may have no obvious signs, there are thousands of cancer cells created in our bodies every single day. The good news is that our immune system takes care of most of them. The bad news is – if we overload our system with toxins, our natural cleansing system cannot do its job properly. And various discomforts, symptoms and diseases start to show up. That is why regular detox is so important nowadays. Even if you don't have any health issues right now, it is a good idea to take a look at these deep cleansing methods and apply them for a short period of time as prevention. If you have any serious illness (including cancer), these detoxes might even save your life. Make sure you consult with your physician and be under medical supervision throughout the process. Make a research on how many people actually managed to cure themselves from this dreadful condition with natural methods. It will lift your spirit and give you the motivation to take your health in your own hands.

The cancer curing detox method by Rudolf Breuss

This healing cleansing method had proven itself extremely effective for thousands of people all over the world. I myself have witnessed a close relative shrinking her brain tumor using this fasting detox. After all it makes a perfect sense – about 80% of our immunity is located in the intestines. And if we nourish our bodies with healthy vegetable juices, we unload our gut from constant digestion, and it starts working full time on healing our tissues.

Fasting and juicing has been used from ancient times to this day. For example, in my country it is an old tradition to have a 3-day complete fasting period (only with water) once a year. But this healing detox has one more positive aspect – it includes lots of vegetable juices, which do not deprive our bodies from nutrients, vitamins, enzymes, anti-oxidants, and so on. No wonder how most ancient healing recipes include fresh fruits and vegetables, roots, and herbs.

This is the same line of thought that brought Rudolf Breuss to developing his magical healing detox method – taking only healing teas and vegetable juices (without the pulp) for a period of time.

Due to this method countless people cured themselves from all types of cancer – breast cancer, colon, cervical, leukemia, prostate, lymphomas, lung, melanomas, brain tumors, bone, liver, throat cancer, etc.

The complete cancer curing program consists of 42 consecutive days taking only fresh juices from roots, vegetables, and drinking pure herbal infusions. That is how we give the immune system time and energy to deal with the health condition.

If you have some other milder health issues, you can apply this method for a short period of time or combine it with light vegan meals as long as you need to. As prevention, you can turn one day of the week or one day of the month into a healing detox with these juices and herbs. People using this program have found a cure for various issues like enlarged prostates, allergies, infertility, and many more. As I have already said – when we strengthen the immune system, it takes care of the impaired tissues and organs by itself.

Breuss's idea was based on the fact that the cancer cells are basically foreign cells. And when we activate the immune system (by taking only liquid vegetable juices), our system destroys and "eats" up everything which is considered not part of our tissues. Through his healing practice over the years and through the personal experience of thousands of people all over the world, his idea stays relevant and adequate to this day.

Let's get to the recipe itself!

The method is very simple to execute, but it requires persistence and dedication. For this healing detox you will need various roots and vegetables – beetroot, carrots, celery root, turnip (preferably the sort with the black skin), and potatoes. The daily quantities are important and they should be as follows:

- *55% **beetroot juice** – 300 ml (10 oz.);*
- *20% **carrot juice** – 100 ml (3.4 oz.);*
- *20% **celery root juice** – 100 ml (3.4 oz.);*
- *3% **potatoes juice** – 10 to 30 ml (0.34-1 oz.) – this is optional;*
- *2 % **black turnip juice** – 10 to 30 ml (0.34-1 oz.).*

Important note: at the beginning start with low amounts of beetroot juice and more carrots. For example, the first day include 50 ml (1.7 oz.) beetroot juice and 350 ml (12 oz.) carrots; the second day – 100 ml (3.4 oz.) beetroots and 300 ml (10 oz.) carrots; the third day – 150 ml (5 oz.) beetroots and 150 ml (5 oz.) carrots, and so on until you reach the above quantities. Beetroot juice is extremely potent and the body needs some time to get used to its strong healing compounds. The potatoes juice can be skipped, except for cases of liver cancer.

Another helpful tip is to start taking the juice mix before beginning the healing detox. This is how the body will slowly get used to the strong taste and effects of the roots. Start with 250 ml (8.5 oz.) a day divided in 3 parts and drink it before each meal. Try to take small sips and really hold it in your mouth to make sure enough saliva is produced. After all, this is a food and it needs proper absorption to take advantage of its healing properties.

Another essential thing to consider when preparing this healing potion is to strain it thoroughly. Use a strainer and cover it with one of two layers of cheesecloth. It is important not to let any pulp remain in the juice. The fiber will load the intestines and they need to be working on healing our bodies 24/7 for this method to be 100% effective.

After you have prepared the juice mixture, pour it into a glass bottle and store it in the fridge. You will be needing it throughout the day.

Start taking this potion from the morning - about 15 – 20 small sips and "chew" it for a while. The saliva is important in absorbing the nutrients in this juice. Drink the remaining liquid throughout the day in small portions. You can add more carrot juice if you like, but the overall quantity should be not more than half a liter a day.

In case you feel extremely hungry, Rudolf Breuss prescribes taking a simple vegetable bullion. The recipe is also very simple – take one onion bulb, dice it and fry it with one tablespoon vegetable oil until it becomes golden brown. You can add other vegetables according to the season and your taste. Next, add half liter pure (2 cups) water and boil it until the vegetables are well cooked. The important part is to strain the soup well, so that it remains only pure and clear liquid. Divide the bullion in 3 – 4 daily portions.

After the healing period is over (42 days), the next step is to reintroduce solid food in our diet. ***This part is extremely important and should not be overlooked or skipped.*** The digestive system had been resting for over a month and we need to be very gentle when activating it. Start adding each of the following food groups for at least 2-3 days or as long as you feel comfortable. Pace yourself!

1. **Sour fruits** – apples, citruses like lemons, oranges, grapefruits, etc.
2. **Starchy fruits** – bananas, medlars, dates, jujubes, etc.
3. **Non-starchy vegetables** – fresh or steamed.
4. **Cereals** – buckwheat, rice, einkorn, millet, etc. As you start adding this food category, remember to follow the food combining principles. For example, do not mix sour foods and carbohydrates like rice and tomatoes.
5. **Flour products**, potatoes, corn powder products, etc.
6. **Legumes** – beans, lentils, peas, chickpeas, and so on.
7. **Seeds and oils** – sesame, sunflower, tahini, etc.
8. **Proteins** – eggs, dairy products, fish, and meat.

If you accidentally make a dietary mistake or rush into the introduction period, the body might react negatively. The main symptoms are bloating and water retention. What you can do is stall the process (eat the foods you have included) and drink field horsetail tea for the next few days. Another option is to take one day and eat only boiled rice (without salt) – it will absorb the excess water in the body.

These are the main points in the healing process according to the Rudolf Breuss system. In the next paragraphs you can find an extended version of this method developed by a Bulgarian healer and physiotherapist.

Cancer curing detox – extended Bulgarian variation

This is an extremely potent cancer (and not only cancer) healing program by an old Bulgarian healer called Vladimir Boshnakov. I want to take some time to tell his story, because it can serve as a perfect example how you can heal and change your life at any point and in any given circumstances. I hope this will give you the motivation and courage to deal with whatever health condition you are dealing with. And for those of you reading this, who just want to use this book as a prevention tool, you may also find lots of useful tips and information to improve the quality of your life.

So, a brief introduction – in 1998 grandpa Vlado found he had 4 incurable illnesses – poor blood circulation to the brain, absolute arrhythmia, ischemic heart disease, and a 76 mm (3 inch) prostate tumor. After a long period of conventional medical treatment with chemotherapy and lots of drugs, his condition further deteriorated. So, he decided to dive deep into the naturopathic knowledge of well-known healers like the famous Bulgarian herbalist Peter Dimkov, the Austrian healing genius Maria Treben, and of course Rudolf Breuss. Combining all this valuable information, he developed and created his own healing method with vegetable juices and herbs. Here I will share with you his method and I hope it will be your powerful assistant in restoring your health and wellbeing!

The base for this detox is the same root juice mix from the Rudolf Breuss' method. Again, it is advisable to start taking the juice before beginning the healing detox itself.

Here we add some herbal infusions in addition to the vegetable juices:

1. **Salvia (Salvia officinalis)** – take 2 tsps. of the herb and mix them with half a liter pure water. Bring the water to boil and let it simmer for 3 minutes. Strain the tea carefully. Next, add 1 tsp. St. John's wort (Hypericum perforatum), 1 tsp. Melissa (Melissa officinalis), and 1 tsp. Mint (Menta piperita) and soak them in the infusion for 10 minutes. After that, just strain diligently so that the plants are completely removed from the water. This tea is extremely powerful and can be used for prevention as well.

2. **Tea for the kidneys** – prepare the following herbal mixture: 15 gr. (3 tsps.) field horsetail (Equisetum arvense), 10 gr. (2 tsps.) "young" spring Stinging nettle (Urtica dioica), 8 gr. (1 1/2 tsp.) common knotgrass (Poligonum aviculare), 6 gr. (1 tsp.) St. John's Wort (Hypericum perforatum). These quantities are estimated for about 3-week period. This powerful herbal mixture is not suitable for long periods of time.

   How to prepare it? Just take a big pinch (half a tablespoon) of the herbal mixture and soak it in a cup of hot water (250 ml) for 10 minutes. Strain the infusion, but don't throw away the herbs. Put them in 2 cups of water and boil it for 10 minutes. Next, strain the decoction and mix both teas – the infusion and the decoction.

If you are wondering why the preparation seems so odd, the explanation is simple. Some of the healing compounds of the herbs can be extracted by infusion. If we boil them, these chemicals will break down and we won't take advantage of their healing properties. On the other hand, there is one more compound we can extract from these plants, but only by boiling - silicic acid. This acid is extremely important and effective when dealing with cancer cells.

This dosage will be enough for 2 days of the healing detox program. Make sure you prepare it the day before because it has to be taken cold on an empty stomach. The daily quantities are 125 ml (4 oz.) of the tea 3 times a day before a meal. As I have already mentioned, this tea is not suitable for long periods of time. Take it according to the schedule for 3 weeks straight. After that, substitute it with calendula infusion for the rest of the treatment.

3. **Bloody Geranium tea (Geranium sanguineum)** – if you can't find this herb in your herbal and bio stores, you can substitute it with Herb-Robert (Geranium robertianum) they have very similar healing effects. Take one pinch of the plant and soak it in hot water for 10 minute, and strain the infusion. This is the daily amount – take it 2-3 times a day in large gulps. Since this herb contains some Radium, it is extremely beneficial for people who are ongoing or who already went through radiation therapy.

4. **Calendula tea (Calendula officinalis)** – as you may recall from the recipe for the kidney tea, calendula infusion is prepared after the 3 weeks of the treatment. Just take 3 tsps. of the herb, soak it in 750 ml (25 oz.) hot water for 3 minutes, and strain the infusion. This is the dosage for 2 days. Take 125 ml (4 oz.) of the tea 3 times a day on an empty stomach.

Here is an example schedule you can follow to help you get a clear picture of the system:

1. 08:00 AM – take 125 ml (4 oz.) of the cold kidney tea on an empty stomach;
2. 08:30 AM – take 125 ml (4 oz.) of the Salvia herbal mix;
3. 09:00 AM – slowly drink and "chew" 125 ml (or less) of the vegetable juice in small sips;
4. 09:30 AM – take 125 ml lukewarm Salvia tea mixture;
5. 10:00 AM – take 125 ml of the juices;
6. 12:00 PM – drink one portion (125 ml) of the kidney tea on an empty stomach;
7. 13:00 PM – take the juice mix again;
8. 17:00 PM – take 125 ml onion bullion, especially if you feel weak and lack proteins;
9. From 18:00 PM to 20:00 PM – drink the last portion of the daily root juice mix;
10. Before going to bed drink 125 ml kidney tea.
11. Choose 2-3 times during the day when you can take a few gulps of the Geranium tea.

Important guidelines:

- *Do not put any sugar or other sweeteners in the teas and the juice;*
- *Do not strain yourself with hard exercises.* This is not an extreme weight loss program. Although naturally the body will shred a couple of pounds, you will regain them quickly after you start reintroducing the foods when the detox is over. Just take walks outside or do some light easy yoga poses.
- *Consult with your doctor about the natural healing detox method you are going to do.* Especially for severe health cases you may need medical surveillance. For example, the blood pressure has to be checked every day and the blood sugar level may fluctuate.
- *During this powerful cleanse you will lose weight.* Your physician needs to track your condition and if you feel extremely weak or unwell, you might want to stop the process. You can resume the detox after you have strengthened your body enough. If everything goes according to plan, after finishing the program you will regain your natural physique.
- *The strengthening regime (if you stopped the detox prematurely) consists of taking the teas and root juice along with some healthy foods described below.*
- *Don't rush to stop taking the vegetable juice after the 42 days are over.* Continue taking small daily dosages for a week or two (on an empty stomach in small sips).

- *Again, do not start eating all food groups at once after the detox.* Reintroduce different meals slowly and gently for a couple of days each.
- *If you experience constipation during the detox, you can take some gentle laxative teas (more about teas at the end of the book),* or take 1 Tbsp. of extra virgin olive oil on an empty stomach 3 times a day, or do a Chamomile enema as a last resort.
- *If you have any heart conditions, consult with your physician before doing the detox.* If you decide to do the cleansing healing program, you can take Hawthorn tincture – 20-40 drops according to you weight.
- *Grandpa Vlado advises us to avoid drinking plain water during this detox.* Instead you can add different herbal infusions according to the specific health issue (see below).

Additional teas according to your condition

You can add more types of teas and infusions in addition to the main recipe as follows:

- **For brain tumors** – the daily dose is 1-2 cups of lukewarm Melissa (Melissa officinalis) tea on an empty stomach. Take in small sips. The dosage is one pinch of the herbal powder boiled for 10 minutes in 150 ml (5 oz.) water.
- **For the eyes** – take one pinch of the herb Eyebright (Euphrasia officinalis) and soak it for 10 minutes in one cup of hot water. This is the daily dosage. Again, drink the lukewarm tea slowly on an empty stomach.

- **For breast, uterus, or ovaries cancer** – to prepare the daily dose – take one pinch of Lady's mantle (Alchemilla vulgaris) and one pinch of Stinging nettle (Urtica dioica) and soak it in 125 ml (4 oz.) hot water for 10 minutes. Take it lukewarm on an empty stomach.
- **For mouth cancer (palate, lips, tongue, tonsils and larynx)** – the herb is anise (Pimpinella anisum). The directions are the same as the previous teas.
- **For skin cancer** – if the moles are smaller than 1 cm (0.4 inch) in diameter, rub them with Greater Celandine (Chelidonium majus) tincture. If they are bigger, rub the skin around the moles, instead of the cancer parts themselves.
- **For bone and lung cancer, or tuberculosis** – the directions for preparing the tea are the same and the herbs are Narrowleaf Plantain (Plantago lanceolata), Lungwort (Pulmonaria officinalis), Ground Ivy (Glechoma hederacea), Mullein (Verbascum), or Fennel (Foeniculum vulgare). Don't worry if you can't find them all – just add the ones you have. The recipe is the same as the above described infusions. You can drink this herbal mix as much as you like, but without any sugar. In cases of tuberculosis, add 1 tsp. Plantago seeds to the mix.
- **For liver cancer** – 2 cups of warm potato peels decoction. If you feel repulsed from this tea, do not take it – the body always gives us signals what it needs, and what it does not. The

additional thing you can add to your healing routine is poultice. Soak some horsetail herb in hot water. Then take the moist herb and place it in a clean cotton cloth. Place the cloth on top of the liver area and tie it with a bandage. Let it sit overnight.

- **For stomach cancer** – take one pinch of wormwood (Artemisia absinthium) or Common Centuary (Centaurium erythraea) and soak it in hot water for 3 minutes. **Don't exceed the amounts of the herbs.** Take this tea lukewarm once a day in small sips. If you have a nervous stomach, take a herbal mix of valerian and wormwood. Take half a teaspoon valerian roots and boil it in 1 cup of water for 3 minutes. Next, pour the decoction on 1 pinch of wormwood and let it soak for 3 minutes.
- **For spleen or pancreas cancer** – drink at least 1 liter (4 cups) of Salvia tea (hot or cold) a day.
- **For leukemia** – in this case you don't need to fast for the 42 days. Take 250 ml (8.5 oz.) of the vegetable juice 3 times a day on an empty stomach. Remember to "chew" it well to produce enough saliva. Eat light vegetarian meals. Don't eat meat, sugar, white flour products, or anything with artificial coloring and preservatives. During the first 2 days drink the kidney tea, and the next 21 days – the Calendula tea. **Important: make sure your home is clean from harsh chemicals (for example naphthalene, chlorine) or other**

common poisons. This rule, of course should be followed by everyone.

Don't forget to slowly reintroduce all food groups after the detox. See the example from the previous point. This process needs to be at least one month. After the healing program is over, it is best to follow some common healthy guidelines – eliminate the toxins from your lifestyle, exercise moderately, have a clean diet, and work on your emotional and spiritual wellbeing.

Here are some helpful guidelines. These can be applied during the detox if your body is not strong enough to fast for 42 days.

1. *Do not eat meat or meat products;*
2. *No sugar, including brown sugar and artificial sweeteners (aspartame, acesulfame K, etc.);*
3. *No fried, smoked, canned, or too salty foods;*
4. *No dairy products* – milk, cream, cheese, butter, and so on;
5. *No alcohol, sodas, or store bought juices;*
6. *No smoking, of course;*
7. *And no coffee or energy drinks;*
8. *Take oats, seeds, legumes, and raw soaked nuts* – buckwheat (the ultimate cancer cell killer), raw apricot seeds, almonds, walnuts, hazelnuts, beans, lentils, boiled or baked potatoes, wholegrain bread, sprouts, and so on;
9. *Take fresh fruits and vegetables* – apples, kiwi, pomegranate, watermelon, melon, pumpkin, strawberries, raspberries, blackberries, tomatoes, red and green peppers, all kinds of cabbage, spinach, carrots, celery, turnip, etc.

10. *Include cold pressed oils* – sunflower, extra virgin olive oil, sesame oil, pumpkin seed oil, etc.
11. *Include herbal infusions* – Salvia, Calendula, Bloody Geranium, Horsetail, Stinging Nettle, St. John's Wort, Melissa, Peppermint, Knotgrass, Green tea, and the onion bullion.
12. *Low fat goat or cow yogurt is also allowed.*

One more thing we should remember, because it is important – avoid being constipated. If your bowels slow down their work, the toxins and poisons will be reabsorbed in the intestines. Take laxative foods (prunes, apples, figs), teas, or make herbal enemas with Chamomile.

There is one last part of this deep detoxing and healing program, which is optional. This is the herbal poultices with Giant horsetail (Equisetum telmateia). This herb contains much more silicic acid than the normal Horsetail. If you can't find this plant, use the regular Equisetum, but in larger quantities.

Every day take about 20 cm (~8 inch) of the Giant Horsetail's stem (with the needles and leaves). This equals 3 Tbsps. of the dried and crushed herb. Place the herb in 1 1/2 liters (6 cups) pure water and bring it to boil. Let the decoction simmer on low heat for 15 minutes. Next, let it soak until the tea cools off to room temperature and strain it with fine strainer or cheesecloth. Divide the liquid in two parts – 1 liter (4 cups) for the poultice, and half a liter for drinking. Make 3 poultices on top of the area of the impaired organ – one in the morning (for 2 hours), one in the afternoon (again for 2 hours), and the last one is before going to bed and stay with it the whole night. You can use a cotton towel – soak it thoroughly in the decoction and squeeze so it does not run, place a plastic foil on top of it and tie it with a comfortable elastic bandage. The poultice does not have to hinder your movement or squeeze you too tight.

I hope this method would help anyone suffering from any type of cancer or serious ailment.

Apitherapeutic Cancer Healing Recipe

The miraculous stories of people who healed themselves from this insidious disease do not end with Grandpa Vlado. I am going to share with you a little known story about a person who managed to beat this illness in the last stage! Let's jump to the beautiful Balkan country of Croatia where Ante Kresic still lives to this day (surprisingly to the doctors). Many years ago in 2001, Ante was shocked by these same physicians who told him he had only a few months to live. He was diagnosed with lung cancer in the last stage. Ante was released from the hospital on April feeling hopeless and powerless. But thankfully, a friend of his shared a miraculous recipe, which had the power to heal and restore the human body. Ante had nothing to lose, so he rushed to prepare the honey mixture to see if it worked. And, oh boy, how it worked! Just several months later the Croatian was already feeling like a different person. And the blood tests confirmed his positive sensations – the cancer was gone! Needless to say the doctors were shocked. Cases like this had been considered "unexplainable miracles". But we have the explanation – honey and other natural herbs and roots have the enormous power to recover our tissues and bring us back to life and vitality.

If you are eager to find out about the recipe is, read on.

Apitherapeutic Cancer Healing Recipe

Ingredients:

- o *500 grams (2 cups) pure, raw unpasteurized* ***honey*** *(preferably Manuka or acacia);*
- o *Some young* ***pine needles*** *(while they are still soft) – adjust the quantity according to the volume of the honey;*
- o *2* ***lemons;***
- o *30 grams (6 tsps.)* ***Turmeric powder;***
- o *500 grams (2 cups)* ***ginger root;***
- o *Some* ***Ceylon cinnamon*** *according to your taste (optional)*

Directions:

1. First we will make the pine needle honey infusion. Take the fresh pine needles and wash them thoroughly. Let them dry well on a towel.
2. Finely grind the needles in a coffee grinder.
3. Mix the ground pine needles with the honey and stir well (with a wooden spoon).
4. Place the mixture in the fridge for 2 weeks.
5. After the honey infusion is ready, we can start preparing the other ingredients. Squeeze the juice out of the lemons and peel and grind the ginger root.
6. Add the lemon juice, the turmeric powder, the ginger paste, and the cinnamon (if desired) in the honey jar, and stir well (with a non-metal utensil).
7. The healing honey mixture is ready.

Take 1 tsp. of the mixture 3 times a day 20-30 minutes before each meal (on an empty stomach). If your body reacts positively from this recipe, you can increase the amount, but don't exceed the daily quantity of 6 tsps.

This apitherapeutic remedy is an excellent prevention option that will strengthen your immune system and guard you against viruses, bacteria, and fungi. It is a perfect addition to your annual preparation for the winter season!

Important note: when using this recipe for healing purposes don't forget to follow the healthy diet guidelines for people with serious illnesses.

Also, it is best to test if you have any bee product allergy or high blood sugar level before implementing this natural healing remedy!

Anti-cancer Remedy with Black Cumin

I am going to share with you the interesting and miraculous healing story of Mila from my homeland – Bulgaria. She was diagnosed with skin cancer and the surgery was inevitable. The operation was urgent and scheduled for only 10 days after the test results confirmed her mole was malignant. In the meantime, Mila decided to try some natural therapies to boost her immunity, and prevent from further cancer cells development on the skin. She was advised to try the healing powers of Black Cumin oil (Nigella Sativa) and Apricot kernel oil. After 10 days of strictly taking the recommended doses of the oils (see below for more details), she anxiously headed towards the operating table. But to her and to the doctor's surprise – the cancer formation was completely gone.

But why were these simple remedies so effective in merely 10 days?

Black cumin contains lots of nutrients and active substances, which are responsible for its healing powers and immune boosting properties. Nigella Sativa is rich in essential fatty acids, niacin, proteins, folic acid, calcium, zinc, iron, phosphorus, thiamine, riboflavin, pyridoxine, carotene, arginine, etc. The arginine is a special compound that helps people with all kinds of traumas, burns and inflammations. It counteracts the free radicals, stimulates the growth hormones secretion and the collagen synthesis, which makes the oil excellent for natural anti-aging therapies. Black cumin also contains another very special chemical called Nigelon. It is extremely valuable for treating respiratory issues like bronchitis and asthma. Nigelon soothes and dilates the bronchi, and suppresses the histamines secretion. (Too much histamine in our blood stream loads the body and leads to histamine intolerance with some pretty uncomfortable symptoms. That is why we need to make sure these compounds are at their normal healthy levels.)

Nigella Sativa is a proven immune booster – it stimulates the thymus – a gland which plays an important role in our natural defense mechanisms. These little precious black seeds have an extremely beneficial effect on the spinal cord. This makes Black cumin a very good natural assistant in dealing with serious diseases like cancer – ideal for prevention and suppressing the tumors' growth. This oil also works as a powerful antibiotic, but unlike the synthetic ones, Black cumin does not harm our beneficial colon bacteria and their colonies. It is still very effective against stubborn malevolent bacteria with antibiotic resistance (like the cholera causing bacteria).

As you can see, Nigella Sativa has some very powerful compounds, which means it can be used for treating numerous ailments and health conditions – allergies, the flu, inflammations in the oral cavity, digestive tract issues, diabetes (lowers the blood sugar level), hemophilia, sinusitis, hemorrhoids, prostatitis, psoriasis, alopecia (balding), diarrhea, chronic fatigue and burnout, colon parasites, low bile secretion, etc. As a whole, Black cumin oil has distinct antiviral, antibiotic, anti-fungal, antibacterial, and slightly diuretic properties.

Another good side of this oil is that it can be used topically on the skin. When taken internally and externally on the scalp, it can prevent from premature graying of the hair, hair loss, and to stimulate its growth. You can even add Black Cumin oil in your homemade organic skin care to moisturize your derma and for anti-aging purposes.

And finally here is an interesting quote from an ancient religious book (Sahih Bukhari 7:71:592): "*There is healing in Black Cumin for all diseases except death.*" I think this says it all about the power of this magical plant.

How to take Black cumin oil?

Depending on the condition the dosages vary from 1 tsp. to 1 Tbsp. 1-2 times a day and since this is a very powerful product, follow the guidelines from your physician.

For the purpose of healing and strengthening your immune system, you can use the following scheme – mix 1 tsp. Black cumin oil with 1 tsp. organic honey and take it 2 times a day on an empty stomach.

For daily de-stress and for a good night sleep take 1 Tbsp. Black cumin oil with 1 Tbsp. honey and mix them in a cup of warm tea. Drink the beverage just before bedtime.

Important note: do not exceed the recommended dosages! This oil is not suitable for pregnant/breastfeeding women, and people with implanted organs. Apply only under medical surveillance.

The other important ingredient in Mila's healing program was Apricot kernel oil. This is also one of Nature's best sources of vitamin B17.

Why is this vitamin so important?

Vitamin B17 is often called "the perfect chemotherapeutic agent", because it selectively destroys only the defected (cancer) cells and keeps the healthy tissue intact. It also boosts the metabolism, slows down aging and works as an analgesic. Apricot kernel oil is also rich in vitamins A, E, F, group B, Omega 6 and 9 fatty acids, etc. They stimulate and amplify many biochemical processes, regenerate the cell membranes and have distinct anti-inflammatory effects. This natural oil is also beneficial for the skin – it stimulates the collagen production and works as organic sunscreen. You can apply this oil to heal from burns and lichens.

The recommended dosage is between 10 to 30 drops of the oil daily – you can add it to your smoothies, juices or salads. For preventive purposes and strengthening the immune system continue taking this oil for 3-6 months. **Do not exceed the recommended quantities!**

Noni – the cancer slayer!

Morinda citrifolia or now mostly known as Noni is a tree mainly found in Asia, South America, The Caribbean, and Polynesia. Recently the fruits of this tree had been discovered to have tremendous positive health benefits for our bodies. It contains large amounts of active substances, such as vitamins (especially vitamin C), microelements, minerals, polysaccharides, polyphenols, flavonoids, iridoids, terpenes, glycosides and alkaloids, such as proxeronine and anthraquinones.

The chemical proxeronine in Noni turns into xeronine once ingested. And xeronine is responsible for stimulating the natural production of endorphins (the "happy" hormones), blocking the feeling of pain and elevating our mood, even causing euphoric sensations. That is why Noni has been considered as an excellent analgesic. But for that painkilling effect to be manifested, xeronine has to be absorbed fully, which happens in the intestines. This means that Noni fruits or extracts have to be taken on an empty stomach to reap their full benefits.

According to the research of Dr. Neil Solomon M.D, Morinda citrifolia can be the key to healing cancer naturally. The plant contains large amounts of polysaccharides and anti-oxidants (even more than Aloe Vera), which strengthen the immune system and stimulate the production of NK cells (our natural "killer" cells). As a result, our bodies remain highly capable of disarming and extracting all newly formed tumors and shrinking larger ones.

Dr. Solomon also claims that Noni can be very effective in stabilizing the blood sugar level and soothing the discomforts related to PMS or enlarged prostate, speeding the tissue recovery from wounds and fighting inflammations.

The benefits of Noni do not end here! This plant is proven to be a powerful detoxifier with strong beautifying effects (especially on the skin). The active substances (such as the terpene called limonene) in Noni normalize the digestion, speed the metabolism, cleanse the blood, the lymph and the intestinal tract. And as we know, our skin is like a mirror to the function of the internal organs, especially the liver and intestines. If we detox and purify these precious organs, our skin glows and clears from acne and pimples.

Noni also contains a certain amounts of Selenium and methylsulfonylmethane (MSM) which is a natural source of Sulfur ("the beauty mineral") – it helps the synthesis of collagen and keratin.

This strange looking fruit has a lot more to offer! It has distinct toning and energizing effects (without any caffeine), antimicrobial, and anti-fungal effects – Noni has been proven to successfully fight skin conditions like eczemas, and various types of infections such as Candida, bone spurs (in combination with physiotherapy), high blood pressure, Osteoarthritis, and chronic fatigue.

Note: consult with your physician before treating yourself with this powerful fruit. It is considered safe, but you need to be extra cautious in case you are pregnant, breastfeeding, or have any serious chronic illness, like liver damage, kidney issues, diabetes, or an allergy to some of Noni's substances.

Doses: depending on the type of extract you are using, the dosages may vary. The general rule is to start with small quantities and slowly increase them over time until you reach 60-70 ml (4-5 Tbsps.) concentrated juice a day. The best way to take the liquid is on an empty stomach mixed with water, coconut water or citrus juice.

Noni works perfectly in combination with Aloe Vera! Which leads us to the next powerful healing recipe:

Aloe Vera & Noni Smoothie

Ingredients:
2 Tbsps. **Aloe Vera gel**
2 Tbsps. **Noni juice**
1 cup **fresh pineapple** (diced)
1 cup **fresh apples** (diced)
2 Tbsps. **coconut milk**

Directions:
Place all ingredients in a blender and mix well. And that's it!
Enjoy!

The Ancient Tibetan Healing Detox

Tibet is a mystical land which still baffles us with its ancient healing and spiritual secrets. One of these is the magical "Tibetan youth recipe". It is designed and used to heal our bodies, boost our immune system, detox us, cleanse all tissues and cells, stimulate the metabolism, shred some extra fat, and keep us young and vital as long as possible. All systems in our body react positively to this natural cure, especially the blood vessels. Even the traditional medicine confirms this magical Tibetan recipe cleanses the arteries and strengthens the blood vessels' walls. Many people around the world who found and tried this ancient treatment managed to cure themselves from some serious diseases and get back their wellbeing. This elixir had been used strictly by the Tibetan monks in order for them to endure and survive in the harsh conditions in the mountains.

The recipe

The recipe for this magical healing detoxifier is very simple. It contains only 2 ingredients – garlic and alcohol. We are going to make a powerful garlic tincture that will rejuvenate, cleanse, and strengthen our body.

Take 350 grams (1 1/2 cup) garlic and mash it until it becomes a homogenous puree. The garlic has to be as fresh as possible – not older than 4 months after it had been harvested. Avoid using metal utensils and containers. Place the puree in a glass sealable jar and try to get the most of the juice from the garlic. Fill the jar with 200 ml. (~ 1 cup) strong alcohol and seal the container. Wrap the jar with some paper to prevent it from light exposure. Place the container in a cool dark place for 10 days. After the time is up, strain the mixture (you can use cheesecloth or a fine strainer) and put the tincture in a glass container. It will be most comfortable for you to put it in a special tincture bottle – it has a dark brown color and a convenient droplet. If you want to take a step further in preparing this wonderful detoxifier, you can use the phases of the Moon. Start the preparation during the New Moon and the tincture will be ready for the Full Moon period.

How to take the Tibetan drops?

This is an essential part of the cleansing and healing program. This recipe is extremely powerful and the body needs to get used to its potent components. Therefore you have to follow a strict schedule. For best results from this tincture use milk to dilute it. The best option, of course, is fresh organic milk from grass-fed goats (or cows) not treated with chemicals and antibiotics. This is not always possible, so take the best quality milk you can find. The quantity is approximately 50 ml (3 Tbsps.) milk for each dosage Tibetan drops. Here is the schedule for the drops themselves:

Day 1: *take 2 drops in the morning, 2 drops at lunch, and 3 drops in the evening;*
Day 2: *4 drops in the morning, 5 drops at lunch, and 6 drops in the evening;*
Day 3: *7 drops in the morning, 7 drops at lunch, and 9 drops in the evening;*
Day 4: *10 drops in the morning, 11 drops at lunch, and 12 drops in the evening;*
Day 5: *13 drops in the morning, 14 drops at lunch, and 15 drops in the evening;*
Day 6: *16 drops in the morning, 17 drops at lunch, and 18 drops in the evening;*
Day 7: *19 drops in the morning, 20 drops at lunch, and 21 drops in the evening;*
Day 8: *22 drops in the morning, 23 drops at lunch, and 24 drops in the evening;*
Day 9: *25 drops in the morning, 24 drops at lunch, and 23 drops in the evening;*
Day 10: *22 drops in the morning, 21 drops at lunch, and 20 drops in the evening;*
Day 11: *19 drops in the morning, 18 drops at lunch, and 17 drops in the evening;*
Day 12: *16 drops in the morning, 15 drops at lunch, and 14 drops in the evening;*

***Day 13:** 13 drops in the morning, 12 drops at lunch, and 11 drops in the evening;*
***Day 14:** 10 drops in the morning, 9 drops at lunch, and 8 drops in the evening;*
***Day 15:** 7 drops in the morning, 6 drops at lunch, and 5 drops in the evening;*
***Day 16:** 4 drops in the morning, 3 drops at lunch, and 2 drops in the evening;*
***Day 17:** 2 drops in the morning, 1 drops at lunch, and 1 drops in the evening;*
***From Day 18** until you finish the tincture, take 25 drops in the morning, 25 drops at lunch, and 25 drops in the evening.*

What to expect from this remedy?

Many people around the world had taken these magical Tibetan drops and report wonderful health and beauty results - relieving chronic headaches, joint pain, improved vitality and higher energy levels, smoother and healthier looking skin, and many more. There are even miraculous unbelievable stories from paralyzed people who managed to regain their ability to walk again. It is no wonder, since garlic is a powerful immune stimulator, antibacterial, antifungal, anti-carcinogenic, and natural antibiotic (without harming the beneficial colon bacteria) agent.

Precautions and counter indication

Although this remedy consists of natural ingredients, it has its limitations, which should not be overlooked or underestimated. ***The Tibetan drops are not suitable for pregnant or breastfeeding women, small children (under 18), and people with severe digestion or stomach***

problems – gastritis, ulcers, etc. Keep in mind that the strong detoxing and healing processes from this garlic tincture may cause symptoms like itching, disturbance in the liver and gallbladder, stomach irritation, flushing (especially in the head area). Make sure you consult with your physician in case you have one or more of these signs or if you have garlic intolerance. People with low blood pressure should also be cautious or completely avoid these Tibetan drops. Consult with your doctor to make sure whether you can take the remedy or not.

Do not eat more garlic during the detoxing period. After you finish the full course, you can repeat it in 3-5 years. That's how strong and lasting this remedy is!

Enhanced version with herbs

If we take the basic recipe and add some healing herbs to it we can enhance the power of this natural remedy. By mixing the mighty garlic with plants, which had proven their magical rejuvenating and healing powers, we create an even stronger immune-boosting and anti-aging natural remedy. These herbs are Helichrysum (Helichrysum angustifolium), Chamomile (Matricaria chamomilla), birch buds (Betula pendula leafs), wild strawberry leaf (Fragaria vesca), and St. John's Wort (Hypericum perforatum).

How to prepare it?

Take 100 gr. (1/2 cup) of each herb and 100 gr (1/2 cup) birch buds and grind them. Mix them well and place them in a glass jar with a tight lid. In the evening take 2 Tbsps. of the herbal mix and soak it in hot water for 10 minutes. Next, strain the mixture and let it cool. Divide the liquid in 2 equal parts and place one half in the fridge. You can drink the remaining one with one teaspoon honey (the tea has to be below body temperature). Don't eat or drink anything else after taking this tea. In the morning take the other half of the tea, warm it slightly, add some honey, and drink it 15-20 minutes before breakfast. Repeat the process every day until you finish the herbal mix.

Detox and Immunity Building Herbs

"A cup of tea would restore my normality."
~Douglas Adams

As promised, in this chapter I will share with you a list of herbs you can use to enhance your detoxing procedures and build a strong immunity. These plants are famous for their healing and cleansing properties. Remember, though, herbs may be natural detoxifiers, but they could be more powerful than we suspect. Do not exceed the dosages and the detox period! It is best to consult with a herbal specialist who can devise you a special cleansing, immune boosting and healing blend for your unique case.

Milk Thistle (Silybum marianum) – Milk Thistle is one of the best herbs for detoxing, strengthening the immune system and boosting the liver (and gallbladder). It has also been proven to help the work of the intestines and the reproductive system. This potent plant can help you take out the cholesterol plaques and triglycerides. The magic of this herb comes from its seeds. They contain a substance called silymarin which helps the liver cells to regenerate through the process of protein synthesis. Silymarin is extremely effective even against the most dangerous liver toxins. Milk Thistle contains various beneficial components – fat-soluble vitamins (F,A,D,E), essential micro and macro elements (Zinc, Selenium, Iodine, Boron, Copper, etc.), and much more. This magical plant and its seeds can be used for prevention or in addition to healing many serious liver illnesses like cirrhosis, jaundice, and hepatitis. It is indispensable for detoxing from strong chemical poisoning – with tobacco, alcohol, heavy metals, etc. The spleen and the digestive tract also benefit greatly from this plant. Taking Milk Thistle tea or powder can have a very good effect on the cardiovascular system (against varicose veins and hemorrhoids), the menstrual cycle in women, discomforts in the pelvis and the kidneys. Here is a recap of the countless benefits from Milk Thistle:

- *lowers the cholesterol level and protects the heart;*
- *slows down and decreases the cancer cells formation (in various cancer types – breasts, lungs, cervix, colon, prostate, kidneys, etc.);*
- *recovers the cells from chemotherapy and radiation;*
- *prevents and slows down the development of Alzheimer's disease;*
- *stabilizes the blood sugar levels;*
- *fights the free radicals and slows down the aging process;*
- *protects from sun radiation and other skin issues;*
- *soothes the menopause symptoms;*
- *heals gastrointestinal issues, including constipation;*
- *it stimulates the gall secretion and thus – prevents from gallstones formation;*
- *it even can be used to counteract death cap (Amanita phalloides) poisoning, and much more.*

Whew! It is very hard to point all of the benefits from this unpretentious wild plant! Before taking this herb in any form, consult with your physician or herbalist! This plant is extremely strong and can cause some negative side effects – diarrhea, upset stomach or skin rashes.

Preparation: soak 1 Tbsp. Milk Thistle seeds in 250 ml (1 cup) hot water for about 10 min. If you want to enhance the taste of the tea, you can add a teaspoon Mint and a teaspoon ground Fennel seeds to the herbal mix. Strain and drink throughout the day.

Cat's claw (Uncaria tomentosa) – Cat's claw is a South American liana, which has been used by the natives in their traditional natural medicine for a long time. It has been valued as a powerful immune booster with distinct anti-oxidative properties. Uncaria tomentosa is a very potent plant, which can even be used as an assisting agent in anti-cancer treatments, and for osteo-articular diseases, acute or chronic viral infections, skin conditions, etc. The plant works as an antibacterial, anti-inflammatory, anti-viral, diuretic, and hypotensive (lowers the blood pressure) natural remedy. ***It is important to remember to supply with a high quality Peruvian Cat's Claw, because of its potent benefits. In comparison, the Northern American variation of the plant does not contain such powerful healing properties, and it can even cause some negative side effects on our bodies!***

Preparation: boil 1 Tbsp. of the herb in 1 1/2 cup (400 ml) pure water for 3 minutes. Cover the pot and let the infusion steep for half an hour. Strain the tea and take 5-6 Tbsps. 4 times a day on an empty stomach (30 minutes before a meal).

If you use Cat's Claw tincture, take 50 drops of the solution 2-3 times a day after a meal, diluted in some water, tea or juice.

Echinacea – the plants from the Echinacea family (Echinacea purpurea, Echinacea angustifolia, Echinacea pallida) are famous for their immune boosting properties. Extracts and infusions from this herb have the power to fight viral diseases, infections, fungal contaminations, inflammations, and to stimulate the regeneration of the tissues. Echinacea purifies the blood and the lymph, suppresses the growth of the staphylococci, streptococci, and viruses. Tinctures, infusions, and poultices from this plant are extremely effective for treating wounds, herpes, burns, urinary and respiratory infections, sour throat, coughs, headaches, vaginitis, sinusitis, urticaria and rashes, gingivitis, influenza, otitis, cystitis, stomach ulcers, etc. As we have discussed in the chapter dedicated to the cancer healing detoxes, immunity plays a big role in these treatments. Strong immunity equals less cancer cells in our bodies. In this line of thought, Echinacea can be a powerful ally when dealing with this insidious ailment. The polysaccharides in the herb stimulate the production of a special chemical (secreted by the macrophages), which destroys the tumors (called cancer cell apoptosis).

Preparation: if you use dry Echinacea blossoms and stalks, boil 1 Tbsp. of the herb in 400 ml (1 1/2 cup) water for 3 minutes. Let it soak for 30 minutes and strain the infusion. Divide the tea in 3-4 equal parts and drink them 3-4 times a day 30 minutes before a meal.

If you use dry roots of the herb, boil 2 tsps. in 2 cups water for 20 minutes. Strain the tea and drink in small sips throughout the day.

If you use Echinacea tincture (alcoholic solution), dilute 25 drops in 6 Tbsps. water and drink it 15 minutes before a meal 2 times a day.

Avoid taking Echinacea extracts during pregnancy, breastfeeding, allergy to the herb and in the evening (it tones the body and could lead to insomnia).

Buckthorn (Rhamnus) – as I already mentioned, this herb should be taken seriously and with great caution. The bark of the plant is used for preparing tea for healing constipation, colitis, ulcers, hemorrhoids, flatulence, excess bile production; it cleanses the body, lowers the cholesterol level, fights stress and depression, even enhances the libido. For best healing purposes it is best to use Sea Buckthorn. It is packed with vitamins (A, B, and C), antioxidants, and immune boosters. It could be beneficial for treating asthma, respiratory problems, liver issues, allergies, loss of appetite, fatigue, etc. This herb stimulates the synthesis of natural collagen, thus making the skin smoother and brighter. The bark of the plant should have been dried for at least one year to be suitable for making tea. The fresh plant contains substances, which may cause nausea and vomiting.

Preparation: For each unit of the herb you need 10 units water. For example, 10 grams (2 tsps.) dried Buckthorn bark should be boiled in 100 gr (1/2 cup) hot water. Drink 100 ml (1/2 cup) of this decoction three times a day. As I have already mentioned, keep this healing procedure short. Consult with your physician. ***Important note: this herb is not suitable for pregnant women - it may cause miscarriage!***

For healing purposes (for the liver, or against parasites), use the fresh fruits of the plant – they must be well matured. You can also find oil made from Buckthorn, which also has beneficial effects on the body.

Liquorice (Glycyrrhiza glabra) – the name literally means "sweet root", and for a reason. This herb and its roots are very sweet, but also extremely healthy. It contains a bunch of beneficial compounds, such as flavonoids, amino acids, tannins, Vitamin C, glycosides, and natural sugars. Taking this plant could have a positive effect on many health issues:

- *it fights infections of the upper respiratory tract* (bronchitis, tonsillitis, even pneumonia);
- *soothes the digestive system* (ulcers, gastritis, flatulence, acid reflux, aphtae, and viral herpes);
- *works beneficially on the excretory system* (frequent urinating, constipation, and Addison's disease);
- *helps regulating irregular menstrual cycles*, and soothes menstrual pains and discomforts;
- *helps people with allergies, arthritis, and skin problems*, such as eczemas and psoriasis.
- *Liquorice is considered to be an aphrodisiac for women.*
- *It also suppresses the appetite*, which makes it the perfect weight loss assistant.

People suffering from diabetes must avoid this herb, because of the containing sugar! This plant is also not suitable for pregnant women, and during breastfeeding.

Preparation: pour half liter (2 cups) pure boiling water into 1 Tbsp. minced Liquorice and let it simmer for about 10 min. Next, take it off the hot plate and let it rest and soak well for half an hour. Take 100 ml (1/2 cup) of this tea on an empty stomach up to 3 times a day. Do not exceed the daily dose of this plant and do not take it for long periods of time!

Coriander (Coriandrum sativum) – this is not just a spice for preparing food, it's a powerful healing and cleansing herb. Its magical properties are numerous. Coriander helps the digestive system, even if you have any stomach pains or discomforts. The essential oil in this plant successfully fights these problems. Other benefits for the gastro enteric tract are counteracting flatulence and constipation. Coriander gently stimulates this area and helps it remove all gas and feces. This herb is an excellent healing plant – it has antiseptic, antifungal, and anti-viral properties. Use Coriander tea in cases of salmonella, infections, barley eye (Hordeolum), gastritis, arthritis, hives, acne, respiratory infections, etc. And that's not all! Many studies show this herb's positive effects on treating serious diseases such as pneumonia, Alzheimer's, Parkinson's, diabetes, and high cholesterol levels. Coriander tea is perfect for women suffering from severe menstruation symptoms. This plant has significant cleansing and detoxifying effects – successfully removes heavy metals from the body, and its green leaves, full of chlorophyll, take out the harmful toxins.

Dosage: pour 200 ml (~ 1 cup) hot water on 2 tsps. ground Coriander seeds. Let the infusion sit for an hour. Strain the mixture and take the tea before a meal 3 times a day (for adults). The doses for children should be prescribed by a pediatrician.

Oregano (Origanum vulgare) – this is another famous spice, which is not used as a decoction very often. And this is a huge mistake! Oregano has healing powers we didn't even suspect. Just like Coriander, this herb is a powerful antiseptic, and it can be used for treating all kinds of infections in the body. It is an immune booster; improves the work of the digestive system; people suffering from stubborn coughs, asthma, and rheumatism san also benefit from this plant, because of its abilities to soothe muscle cramps and joint pain. Oregano is packed with antioxidants, vitamins, flavonoids, polyphenols, and other beneficial compounds. This herb is a perfect natural antibiotic (without destroying the beneficial colon bacteria), with strong antifungal, anti-parasitic, antiviral, anti-histamine, and yeast inhibiting properties. Oregano is considered to be very effective even against serious diseases, such as metabolic syndrome, cancer, hypertension, and high cholesterol levels. This plant's powerful compounds prevent the cells from the detrimental oxidative damage, thus keeping them away from chronic illnesses. And these are not all of its magical healing powers! Oregano gently cleanses the body by flushing away toxic debris in the colon, helps people with chronic inflammations, osteoporosis, chronic fatigue, and frequent headaches. This green spice is essential for cancer prevention. Use this plant as morning tea or even better - include this plant fresh in your menu. You can use it as a food supplement for stimulating the bowel movement, but only for short periods of time. ***Take it not more than one month, do not overdose it, and do not take it if you are pregnant or breastfeeding.***

Preparation: pour half a liter (2 cups) hot water on 1 Tbsp. dry Oregano leaves. Let it soak for an hour and strain. Take 1 cup of the infusion 4 times a day before a meal.

Mint/Peppermint (Mentha/Mentha piperita) – you can never go wrong with the classics! Peppermint tea has many benefits for the human body – it relieves daily stress and relaxes the muscle tension; cleanses the sinuses, lungs, and the throat; takes out the toxins from the body and helps us lose weight naturally; stimulates the digestion and fights flatulence, colitis, diarrhea, nausea and constipation. This is an excellent herb for any liver and gall issues. Mint decoction has the same benefits, but it also works as a hormonal regulator for women. It gently stimulates the estrogen production, relieving PMS and menopause symptoms, clearing acne and making the skin smoother. It also decreases female body hair growth when taken regularly.

Preparation: pour half a liter (2 cups) hot water on 2 Tbsps. dry Peppermint leaves. Let it soak for 10 minutes and strain. Take 1 cup of the infusion 3-4 times a day before a meal.

St.John's Wort (Hypericum perforatum) – another magical, powerful, and extremely beneficial plant for daily use. The herb is packed with goodies – flavonoids, polyphenols, naphtodianthrones, phloroglucinols, pseudohypericin, phloroglucinol, essential oil. Its numerous healing properties deserve our attention. Here are some of them: St.John's Wort is one of the most famous natural antidepressants known to man – it soothes anxiety, insomnia, persistent dark thoughts, neurosis, phobias, headaches, migraines, and hysteria. And since the nervous system is tightly connected to the digestion, this plant helps us recover from issues such as gastritis, ulcers, stomach pain and cramps, reflux, and nervous stomach. This plant is a valuable aphrodisiac, because sexual appetite is often disturbed from depression, daily stress, and anxiety. Try this tea if you suffer from sore throat, bronchitis, pleurisy, rhinitis, gout, arthritis, rheumatism, cardio-vascular problems, diarrhea, and many more. St.John's Wort decoctions gently cleanse the body and calm the nerves while detoxing. Its diuretic properties purify the body, stimulate the bowel movement, and support the work of the kidneys. This magical herb also boosts the thyroid, the gall (taking out gallstones), and even helps people recovering from pneumonia. Beside all these benefits from St.John's Wort tea, there are a couple of precautions. This plant is very powerful and it could enhance some medications, or debilitate others. For example, it magnifies the effect from some antidepressants, while disempowers the effectiveness from contraceptives. ***People with hypotension should also be very careful when taking this herb – St.John's Wort may lower the blood pressure. Another thing to consider is photo sensitivity – if you apply this plant regularly, take extra protection measures against UV radiation.*** The herb increases the skin's sensitivity to light. So, before taking this plant, consult with a physician to determine if this yellow herb is suitable for you.

Preparation: put 2 Tbsps. dry herb (with the blossom) in 400 ml (1 1/2 cup) hot water. Boil the mixture for 5 minutes, take it off the heat and let it soak for 30 minutes. Strain the infusion. Take 120 ml (1/2 cup) tea daily, the rest of the decoction put in a fridge (store for not longer than 12 hours).

Chicory (Cichorium intybus) – this is a wonderful plant to start your day with! It is one of the most popular healthy coffee substitutes. Chicory contains many beneficial substances, which improve our health – Calcium, Phosphorus, Iron, Magnesium, Vitamins A1, B1, B2, C, E. It is suitable for people with diabetes, because of its low sugar content (there are only 4 g carbohydrates in 100 g Chicory). The special thing about this plant is the containing compound called inulin. This is a polysaccharide, which has a powerful beneficial effect on our organism. It is a natural prebiotic (stimulates the growth of the good colon bacteria). This makes Chicory a gentle, but very effective immune stimulator (the colon flora is responsible for around 80% of our immune system). But there is more! Inulin takes toxic metabolites out of our system, lowers the blood pressure, lowers the cholesterol and triglycerides levels in the liver, stimulates the bowel movement (without making the intestines lazy), lowers the blood sugar level, enhances the lipid metabolism for people with Diabetes type 2, helps us absorb more minerals from our nutrition, and many more. Chicory has been proven throughout the years for being extremely beneficial for the digestive system. It stimulates the bowel movement, cleanses the blood, and strengthens the immune system during the flu and colds. This plant is also valuable for the heart – it counteracts the malevolent effects of fats and alcohol on the cardiovascular system. Chicory tea/coffee tones the body while soothing the nervous system, and fights daily stress.

Preparation: pour 200 ml (1 cup) hot water on 2 tsps. ground dry Chicory root. Let it sit for an hour and strain. This is the daily amount – divide it into 4 equal parts and take before a meal.

Thyme (Thymus vulgaris) – this one of the best herbs to start your day with and to include in your gentle detox. It contains several types of antioxidants (flavonoids, terpinene, beta carotene), which fight the free radicals, preserving our cells from degeneration and aging. Thyme also has a special compound called thymol, which has a strong antimicrobial effect – it destroys different kinds of pathogenic microorganisms – viruses, fungi, parasites, bacteria. Many medical surveys state that Thyme can counteract one of the most common causes of fungal infections – Candida fungi. Because of these antiseptic properties, Thyme is frequently used in different products for oral health – it prevents from plaque deposition. This herb is very effective for a number of problems connected to the respiratory tract – cough, asthma, bronchitis, croup, tonsillitis. Thyme tea is excellent for healing diarrhea, flatulence, rheumatoid diseases, and parasites, such as the hookworm (a parasite found in the duodenum and the small intestine). Some herb experts state that Thyme is effective against headaches, high cholesterol, high temperature, and discomforts from liver diseases.

Preparation: soak 1 tsp. dry Thyme in 250 ml (1 cup) hot water for 30 minutes. Strain the mixture and drink in the next 12 hours.

Melissa (Melissa officinalis) – this herb is another excellent healthy alternative for the morning coffee. Its flavor reminds us of lemon, and it's as beneficial as the citrus fruit. It has proven its antibacterial, antioxidant, analgesic, and spasmolytic properties. There are many health issues, which can be soothed with this plant. Such as Alzheimer's, migraine, insomnia, anxiety, stomach pain and cramps, colitis, high temperature, heart problems, menstrual disorders, menopausal discomforts, issues with the thyroid gland, skin inflammations, gout, catarrh, herpes, nausea (even caused by pregnancy), toothaches, arthritis, and rheumatism. As you can see Melissa has a wide variety of healing properties. It has proven itself effective even for some cases of depression, tinnitus, Hashimoto, and hyperthyroidism. Another good side of this herb is its gentle female hormone balancing effect. That's why it is known as the "feminine herb". Regular consumption of Melissa tea can detox the body, take out all excess water, stimulate the metabolism, decrease the cellulite under the skin, and enhance weight loss.

People diagnosed with epilepsy or brain damages should consult with a doctor before taking Melissa on a daily basis. This herbal tea is also not recommended for pregnant women, for people with severe intestine and stomach infections, severe coughs, and liver diseases.

Preparation: soak 1 Tbsp. dry Melissa leaves in 400 ml (1 1/2 cup) hot water for 20 minutes. Strain the mixture and drink in the next 12 hours.

Cranberry (Oxycoccus) – this fruit is famous for its healthy effects on our bodies. It is mainly used for treating infections of the urinary tract. Cranberries are one of the biggest natural sources of Vitamin C, which makes them perfect for the flu season. They also have strong diuretic and disinfecting properties and can be used for treating kidney stones, gout, rheumatism, pyelonephritis, and cystitis. You can use it as fruit tea or as fresh juice. The juice option is preferred when treating issues with the upper respiratory tract. Cranberries are full of antioxidants, which makes them perfect for slowing the aging process and counteracting neuro-degenerative diseases, such as Alzheimer's. They also lower the blood pressure and protect the cells from damages of free radicals. You will find all kinds of good stuff in these tiny fruits – vitamins, minerals, microelements, flavonoids, essential fatty acids (Omega 3 alpha-linoleic and Omega 6 linoleic acids), carotenoids, and phytosterols. These precious red fruits have been proven to dissolve the plaque on our teeth, kill bacteria in the mouth, and last, but not least – Cranberries are powerful anticancer natural remedy.

Preparation: soak 2 Tbsps. dry cranberry fruits in half a liter (2 cups) hot water. Let it sit for an hour and strain. Divide into 3-4 parts and take before a meal.

Stinging Nettle (Urtica dioica) – this is one of the most beneficial healing herbs known to men. Consider choosing this plant if you want to boost your natural blood production process. People with anemia or hemorrhages can benefit immensely from Stinging Nettle. This tea is excellent for refreshment and toning during spring fatigue. This magical plant is full of essential compounds for our bodies – Silicon, Potassium, Calcium, proteins, Iron, Sulfur, essential oils, amino acids, formic acid, and many more. Stinging Nettle roots contain a lot of life sustaining substances – water concoction from this plant can boost the organism and sooth health issues such as slow metabolism, diabetes, rheumatism, asthma, headache, fever, jaundice, cough, skin conditions, lymph inflammation, etc. Taking this herb as tea, cooked meal, or fresh smoothie can significantly vitalize the exhausted body; stimulate the bowel movement, detox, and fight vitamin deficiency. Be cautious when taking this herb for longer periods, and avoid overdosing, because it may irritate the stomach.

Preparation: soak 2 Tbsps. Stinging nettle leaves in 400 ml (1 1/2 cup) hot water for an hour. Strain and take 120 ml (1/2 cup) of the tea daily. Store the rest of the tea in the fridge.

The preparation for tea from Stinging nettle roots is the same with just one Tbsp. of the herb instead of 2.

Dandelion (Taraxacum) – Dandelion's leaves contain many important compounds, which are necessary for our bodies – vitamin B6, thiamine, riboflavin, vitamin C, Iron, Calcium, Potassium, folic acid, Magnesium, Manganese, etc. This plant can supply the impressive 535% of the recommended daily dose of vitamin K, and 110% for vitamin A. Some of the flavonoids in this herb (such as zeaxanthin and cryptoxanthin) have acute healing properties. Zeaxanthin protects the retina from the ultraviolet sunrays, while cryptoxanthin boosts the immune response against chemotherapy resistant cancer cell formation (especially in the lungs and mouth). Some of the specific compounds in this plant are inulin (slows down sugar absorption), Tof-CFR (counteracts cancer cells), Lentinan (has an anti-viral effect), pectin (supports the intestines), Apigenin and Luteolin (anti-inflammatory, anti-oxidants, anti-spasmodic), Choline (enhances memory), Gallic Acid (fights diarrhea and bacteria), Linoleic and Linolenic Acid (boost the immune response and the cardiovascular system), Sesquiterpene compounds, Triterpenes, Taraxasterol (stimulate the liver, the gallbladder, the digestive system, and have an anti-fungal effect). As you can see there are so many beneficial substances in one little plant, which make it extremely beneficial. It also has been proven to have anti-cancer properties. A research run by the University of Winsor, Ontario, concludes that a Dandelion root extract stimulates the cancer cell apoptosis (death of the cancer cell) without causing toxicity in our body. And this is just the tip of the iceberg. This plant, although considered to be unwanted weed, can serve a great healing purpose. Dandelion tea can be effective against different health issues – prevention and treating some liver problems; tones the body, works as a delicate laxative; cleanses the blood and the skin; dissolves kidney stones; supports the digestive system; promotes weight loss; prevents and lowers high blood pressure, high blood sugar and cholesterol levels; helps people with anemia; eliminates stomach acidity and flatulence.

Preparation: soak 2 tsps. Dandelion leaves in 200 ml (1 cup) hot water for 30 minutes. Strain and take the infusion in the evening before going to bed.

For Dandelion roots the recipe is bit different. In the evening pour 250 ml (1 cup) hot water on 2 tsps. dry Dandelion roots and let it sit overnight. In the morning strain the infusion and drink throughout the day in 2-3 equal part.

Wild basil (Clinopodium vulgare) – again, this is one little known wild mountain plant with many cleansing and healing properties. The urinary tract benefits immensely from this tea – in cases of cystitis and kidney stones. Women should really consider drinking this decoction for it gently balances the hormones, soothes mastopathy and fights myomas. It also has been proven effective against serious diseases, such as diabetes, Parkinson's, and even cancer. If you combine drinking this tea with topical use in the form of poultice, you may overcome stubborn issues like warts (including ones cause by HPV), dandruff, seborrhea, eczemas, callus, and other skin problems.

Preparation: pour 400 ml (1 1/2 cup) hot water on 1 Tbsp. Wild basil in a sealable container. Put the lid on and let the infusion sit for 1 hour. Strain the mixture and divide it into 3 parts. Take each part before a meal for one day.

Hawthorn (Crataegus) – cleansing the body requires strong cardiovascular system, especially if we decide to include sweating activities in our detox program. Hawthorn is one of the best herbs for supporting the heart – it tones the muscles and the arteries. There is a specific substance in this plant, called proanthocyanidins, which is responsible for the most of the benefits we can reap. Here I will make a short summary – consider including Hawthorn decoction if you want a natural support for treating high blood pressure and high cholesterol levels; atherosclerosis; arrhythmia; angina; ischemic heart disease; cardiac neurosis; insomnia; some cases of headaches (depending on the source of the pain); hyperthyroidism (Graves' disease) – Hawthorn stimulates the normal thyroid function; enlarged prostate; dizziness/vertigo; assists with weight loss and anti-cellulite programs; soothes menstrual pain, and rheumatics, and many more. If you have or suspect you have a serious health condition, or if you take prescription medications, don't forget to consult with your physician how to safely include hawthorn in your healing scheme.

Preparation: take 1 cup pure water and bring it to boil, add 1 tsp. dry Hawthorn fruits and let them simmer for 10 minutes. Take the decoction off the heat and let it soak for 20 more minutes. Strain and take before a meal.

Rooibos (Aspalathus linearis) – this popular tea is one of the best refreshing coffee substitutes. It has tons of benefits and healing compounds. It contains lots of antioxidants, vitamins, and microelements such as Iron, Calcium, Potassium, Copper, Manganese, Zink, and Magnesium. This plant does not contain caffeine, and oxalic acid, which makes it perfect for people prone to kidney stones formation. It also contains just a small amount of tannins, so the tea refreshes you without irritating the nervous system. You can count on Roiibos tea for counteracting headaches, insomnia, asthma, eczemas, weak bones, hypertension, allergies, and slowing down the aging process. This magic herb is valuable for people with diabetes as well. The antioxidant aspalathin regulates the blood sugar level and lowers the insulin resistance. It also has proven its spasmolytic properties – it soothes stomach pains and cramps. People with different types of allergies and respiratory issues can find natural relief from Roiibos tea.

Preparation: soak 1 tsp. Roiibos tea in one cup hot water for 5 minutes. Strain the infusion and drink hot or cold. You can add fruits or lemon juice according to your taste. The best part is you can steep the herb more than once.

Matcha green tea – This is one of the most common healthier alternatives to coffee. If you still need your daily dose of stimulants, at least you can choose this option, which does not drain the Calcium out of your bones. Green tea contains a compound called thein – it is a form of the caffeine, except it is found in tea leaves and it's much healthier. Let's get back to Matcha. In the East, it is called the Royal tea, because of its healing properties and numerous benefits for the body. One of the main reasons is the high amount of chlorophyll, which we ingest with the tea. Unlike other types of herbal decoctions, Matcha is taken with its leaves (ground as a fine powder). And we already know the healing and detoxing power of the green leaves. But Matcha is special, because it is grown in shady places, which enhances the chlorophyll amounts in the leaves of the plant. Here are some other interesting facts about this herb – it contains 6.2 times more antioxidants than Goji berry; 7 times more than natural black chocolate; 17 times more antioxidants than wild blueberries, and the impressive 60.5 times more than the famous spinach. This makes this tea one of the best anti-aging natural remedies. Free radicals are not just responsible for accelerating aging, but also for cancer cells formation. In other words, regular consumption of Matcha tea is an excellent cancer prevention tool. That's not all, the active compounds in this herb counteract the precipitation of the dangerous cholesterol plaques on the blood vessels' walls. Matcha tea has been scientifically proven to boost the metabolism and promote fat burning. This hot beverage can improve your memory, boost your mood, strengthen the immune system, and give you more energy throughout the day.

Preparation: take 1/2 – 1 tsp. Matcha tea powder and place it in a bowl (you can use the traditional Japanese chawan). Take 100-170 ml (1/2 cup) pure water and start slowly pouring it on the green powder while stirring the mixture. For best results you can use the special ritual brush called chasen. When the powder is fully blended with the water and it forms nice gentle foam, the tea is ready for consumption.

White/Green/Black tea (Camellia sinensis) – these are the most common types of tea from ancient times until this day. They have the same healing and refreshing properties like the Matcha type, but in this case we don't ingest the leaves themselves. Actually, there are only 6 types of tea – white, green, yellow, black, oolong, and pu-erh, they are all the same plant (Camellia sinensis), but the processing (fermentation) of the leaves is different. No matter which one you choose, they all have similar beneficial effects for us. Camellia tea is packed with antioxidants – one cup of green tea has more antioxidants than 10 cups of fresh apple juice. The plant is rich in flavonoids and can be a powerful cancer prevention assistant. It also lowers the "bad" cholesterol level, and fights hypertension. This makes it perfect for protecting the heart from various issues. Green tea (or any other type of tea from Camellia leaves) has been proven to strengthen the bones, teeth, gum, and boost the immune system. It has antibacterial, antiviral properties, and balances the blood sugar level. The skin also benefits from this beverage – green tea protects it from the free radicals, keeping it strong and youthful.

Preparation:

Black tea – soak 3 tsps. in 200 ml (1 cup) hot water for 5 minutes and strain.

Green tea – first boil 200 ml (1 cup) pure water and let it cool off to 70-80 degrees Celsius (158-176 F). Pour the hot water on 3-4 tsps. Green tea and let it soak for 2-3 minutes.

White tea – boil a cup of pure water and wait until it cools off just a little bit (to about 90 degrees Celsius/194 F). Steep some of the white tea leaves in the water for 1-2 minutes.

Speedwell (Veronica) – this is another little know plant, which can beautifully assist you in your detox and healing program. Here is what this herb can do for you! Speedwell is best known for its abilities to effectively lower the high blood pressure. It also cleanses the lungs – helps you cough out excess mucus and soothe bronchitis and asthma. Veronica tea removes all the tiny kidney stones, enhances the memory, and fights dizziness. This plant gently lowers the cholesterol levels, supports the nervous system in cases of neurosis or fatigue. You can use it for different types of urinary problems, hoarseness, early stages of tuberculosis, haemoptysis, blood in the urine, etc. Although there are no side effects found from taking Speedwell tea, remember not to self-medicate, especially in cases of serious symptoms!

Preparation: soak 1 Tbsp. Veronica in 2 cups hot water for an hour. Strain and drink throughout the day.

Greater celandine (Chelidonium majus) – this is a very common simple herb that can be found in various places. Although it is considered just a weed, it definitely doesn't deserve to be underestimated. The plant's healing and cleansing properties had been known even from the ancient Greeks. They called it "a gift from God". Today the herb is used mainly as a natural laxative, urinary tract stimulator and a natural garden insecticide. But it does much more than that – Chelidonium can work as a powerful detoxifier and healer. There are medical researches that show how the active substances in this simple common plant can kill cancer cells effectively. It also stimulates the bile production (cleanses the liver and gallbladder), and it has anti-inflammatory and analgesic properties. It can be taken as a complementary drug for hepatitis, cholecystitis, pancreatitis, ulcer, stomach polyposis, colitis, etc. The juice from the plant's roots is an excellent topical cure for all kinds of skin issues - warts, calluses, pimples, eczema, fungus, herpes, etc.

Preparation: steep 1 Tbsp. of the Chelidonium in 400 ml (1 1/2 cup) hot water. Let the infusion cool off and strain. Take 1 Tbsp. of the tea 15 min before a meal 4 times a day.

Do not exceed the dose – the herb becomes toxic in large quantities!

Bearberry (Uvae Ursi) – this wild fruit and its leaves are one of the best healing plants for the urinary tract, but it also works wonders for the intestines. It is a natural immune booster and tones the body as a whole. It contains chemicals called hydrochinons, which have strong antibacterial properties. Some researches state, that bearberry is effective even against bacterial infections caused by Staphylococcus and Escherichia coli. ***When using Bearberry do not overdose, because it may cause nausea, vomiting, fever, and other unpleasant side effects. This tea is also not suitable for pregnant and breastfeeding women, and children under the age of 12.*** When consuming Uvae Ursi tea regularly avoid taking sour foods and drinks, which contain large quantities of Vitamin C. They will lower the healing effect of the plant. Another point to consider is the duration of taking Bearberry – avoid using it more than one week – the containing tannins will accumulate in the body. Too much tannin will have the same negative effects as consuming caffeine on a regular basis – increased nervousness, tremors, Iron and Calcium deficiency.

Preparation: this tea is being prepared a little different. Pour half a liter (2 cups) cold water on 1 Tbsp. Bearberry leaves and soak them for 8-10 hours at room temperature. Next, put it on the stove and boil for 5 minutes. Strain the infusion and drink 100 ml (1/2 cup) of the tea daily. Store the rest of the tea in the fridge.

Hop cones (Humulus lupulus) – when you hear hop, you may think of beer. But did you know you can have a cup of tea from these cones, which will help you detox, cleanse the colon, and fight constipation? Due to some of its beneficial compounds (such as flavonoids, herniarin, dicumarinum, umbelliferone, bitter substances, essential oils), it has many other healing properties – it cleanses the blood and helps people with anemia; supports the nervous system – soothes menopausal discomforts, alcoholic delirium, hysteria, insomnia, anxiety, neuralgia, etc.; it's an absolute gem for the digestive tract and the intestines – stimulates the healthy levels of appetite, counteracts poor digestion, it is used against stomach cramps, colitis, IBS (irritated bowel syndrome), parasites, and many more; hop cones are excellent for gallbladder and/or bile ducts inflammations; the plant will lower the high body temperature, soothe pain, fight inflammations, and take the toxins out of the body; it is an excellent remedy for kidney stones, liver problems, water retention; it is also suitable for upper respiratory tract issues, such as coughs. Hop cones have antiseptic properties, but they are also a source of phytoestrogen – this should be taken into consideration. ***That is why breastfeeding women should avoid taking this plant, it may decrease the lactation. This herb is also not suitable for people with cardiovascular problems – strokes, heart attack, angina, etc. Avoid large doses of the herb and do not take it for long time intervals.***

Preparation: soak 2 Tbsps. ground dry Hop cones in 400 ml (1 1/2 cup) hot water for 20 minutes. Strain the infusion and drink 100 ml (1/2 cup) of the tea daily. Store the rest of the tea in the fridge.

Corn hair (Stigmata Maydis) - you may hear this for the first time, but corn hair can be used as water decoction to treat constipation and to gently cleanse the body. You will be surprised how many beneficial and healing properties this simple plant contains. Let's start with the contents – Vitamin K, saponins, tannins, fats, sterines, flavonoids, pantothenic acid, and many more. When to apply corn hair tea? This water infusion of the plant is an excellent natural remedy for the urinary tract. And as we know, it is responsible for flushing out toxins and retained extra water. Drink this tea if you have kidney stones, inflammation and/or edema of the urinary tract, bile stagnation, liver and/or gallbladder problems, etc. It also assists people with diabetes, suppresses excessive appetite (helps with weight loss), and soothes the nervous system (especially in cases of atherosclerosis). Corn hair decoction has diuretic properties and it's applicable for uterine bleeding, nose bleeding, and painful menstruation; it is also used in Gynecology for causing contractions. It has antibacterial and antifungal properties against trichophytons and monilia; combined with suitable diet, it assists with lowering the cholesterol levels. ***If you are pregnant and you want to take corn silk tea, consult with your physician first. People with jaundice, thrombophlebitis, and ones who are prone to blood clotting, should avoid this herb!***

Preparation: soak 2 Tbsps. Corn hair in 400 ml (~1 1/2 cup) hot water for 30 minutes. Strain the infusion and take 120 ml (~1/2 cup) daily before a meal.

White Mistletoe (Viscum album) – this famous semi parasitic shrub is packed with important ingredients such as viscotoxin, inositol, flavonoids, tannins, vitamin C, provitamin A, organic acids, proteins, resins, etc. The viscotoxin compound is responsible for the plant's ability to lower the blood pressure and to prevent from vascular cramps by dilating the blood vessels. It also tones the heart muscle, slows down the heart rhythm, and boosts the cardiovascular system as a whole. Anything related to hemorrhages can be treated with White Mistletoe – nose bleeding, bleeding hemorrhoids, uterine hemorrhage, long and heavy menstruation, etc. Other interesting benefits of this plant are counteracting issues like fungal infections, epilepsy, diseases of the nervous system, dizziness, headaches, neuralgias, atherosclerosis, arthrosis, pertussis, edemas, chronic joint problems, enhances the uterine contractions helping women with the natural birth process, stimulates the breast milk production, etc. There are even some scientific and medical researches on the anticancer effect of White Mistletoe.

Preparation: take 300 ml (~1 cup) pure water and bring it to boil. Add 1 Tbsp. White Mistletoe leaves and simmer for 5 minutes. Take it off the heat and let it cool off. Next, strain the infusion and divide it into 3 parts. Take each part after a meal.

Important note: this is one of the herbs, which is not suitable for long use, and should not be overdosed. Also its white fruits should not be digested, for their toxicity.

Horsetail (Equisetum arvense) – this herb contains more than 25 main compounds essential for us humans – vitamin C, silicates, flavonoids (equisetrin, luteolin, isoquercitrin), saponins (equisetonin), beta-carotene, alkaloids (nicotine in extremely small amounts), oxalic acid, tannins, and many more. Horsetail is an excellent source of important microelements – it's rich in natural Silicone, Potassium, Manganese, Sulfur, etc. Why should we consider drinking this plant's decoction? One of the main reasons is the high silicon quantities – this element is commonly found in nature, but our bodies are often in lack of it. If you really want to keep your bones, joints, and ligaments in perfect shape, you should pay extra attention to silicone. It keeps the bones strong, while the connective tissue – elastic. In book 1, we talked about yoga and its wonderful benefits for our holistic health. Well, you can call Horsetail the ultimate "yoga herb"! Conventional medicine states that Silicon enhances our Calcium absorption, while other scientific sources state that once ingested, Silicon itself transmutates into Calcium. It doesn't really matter which statement is true, the important thing is Horsetail can be considered essential for fighting osteoporosis. Ladies pay attention! Natural Silicon is not only good for your bones, but also for the hair, nails, and skin! But let's get back to detoxing. This herb has been known in Chinese natural medicine as an energy booster with strong diuretic properties. It alkalizes the urine and stimulates its production with up to 30%. This makes it good for taking out toxins and fighting urinary infections. Recent Russian studies find that this plant is good for detoxing from lead deposits in the human organism. It also has been found that Horsetail is an excellent natural remedy for recovering the lung tissues from respiratory illnesses, such as tuberculosis. One important note about taking diuretics is the subsequent Potassium deficiency. But when it comes to taking Horsetail, this is not an issue – it has the ability to keep a healthy Potassium-Sodium balance in the body. ***However, this plant is not recommended for children, people with type 2 Diabetes, people who take anticoagulant medications, pregnant and breastfeeding women. Do not overdose this herb!***

Preparation: boil 2 Tbsps. Horsetail in 400 ml (1 1/2 cup) water for 3 minutes. Take it off the heat and let it soak for an hour. Strain the infusion and divide it into 3 parts. Take each part 3 times a day after a meal.

Raspberry leaves (Rubus idaeus) – we all know the deliciousness of the raspberries, but their fruits are not the only healthy part of the plant. Raspberry leaves are extremely beneficial for the human organism and its immunity. The herb is rich in vitamins C, A, D, Potassium, Phosphorus, Calcium, etc. which help us fight against the colds, the flu, and respiratory issues; improve the digestion and soothe the symptoms of gastritis and enteritis; relieve the menstrual and premenstrual cramps, and counteract the infections. Raspberry leaves tea is an excellent healthy beverage for all active athletes, people with anxiety, insomnia, and chronic fatigue. The plant has a gentle detoxing, purifying, and toning effects.

Some precautions: the infusion is not suitable for pregnant women and people with an allergy to the plant. Make an allergy test by taking just one small cup of the tea and wait for several hours to see if there are any negative symptoms!

Preparation: pour 1 cup boiling water on 1 Tbsp. dry crushed raspberry leaves. Cover the container and steep the herb for 10 minutes. Strain the infusion and drink. The maximum daily dose is 1 cup of tea 3 times a day after a meal.

Rest Harrow (Ononis repens) – this is another beautiful healing plant, which Mother Earth has given us. It looks like a wild flower, but don't be fooled by its good looks, it has many beneficial properties. Rest Harrow tea can effectively start your cleansing procedure by taking out all excess water retained in the body, and boost the work of almost every organ and system. One of its magical properties is helping couples with reproductive issues, finally conceive. Rest Harrow is also very effective with taking out gallstones. If you are fighting with excess weight, especially if it is caused by hormonal imbalance, or irregular menstruation cycle, this is the herb for you. Since it gently balances the female hormones, a detoxing program with Rest Harrow can significantly reduce cellulitis and prevent from mastopathy. This is one of the plants, which can be used during pregnancy and breastfeeding in order to protect the breasts. Consult with your doctor beforehand. Don't worry, gentlemen, this plant is suitable for you, too. Drink Rest Harrow roots tea against enlarged prostate. Since this plant has acute diuretic properties, it is perfect for fighting issues of the urinary tract and genitals, especially cystitis and/leucorrhea; also gout, osteophytes (bone spurs), hemorrhoids, varicose veins, constipation, colitis, stomach cramps. This herb is also an anti-inflammatory remedy – use it in case of rheumatism pains. Some researches state that Rest Harrow can be effective even for hypertension and heart failure. ***Do not***

take this herb for long periods of time without medical supervision. Do not overdose. If you notice high stomach acidity, stop drinking this tea. This plant is not suitable for people with thrombophlebitis or other illness connected to clotting.

Preparation: pour half a liter (2 cups) hot water on 3 Tbsps. dry Rest Harrow roots and soak it for 30 minutes. Strain it and drink 100 ml (1/2 cup) of the infusion 3 times a day before a meal. Take this tea not longer than 10 consecutive days. Take a one-week break and repeat the course if needed.

Melilot (Melilotus) – this plant is packed with healing compounds, such as flavonoids, coumarin glycosides, resinous substances, tannins, cholin, mineral salts, essential oil, etc. All these beneficial ingredients can help people suffering from insomnia, anxiety, menopause discomforts, upper respiratory issues, pain in the kidneys, bladder, and intestines, flatulence, increased blood clotting, migraines, hypertension and its consequences, increases lactation for breastfeeding women, against hemorrhoids, varicose veins, PMS, edemas, gout, coronary artery disease, recovery of liver tissues, tympanum inflammation, and many more. WOW! So many benefits from a single plant! There is one downside, though – ***this herb is not suitable for long term use and should be taken under medical supervision. Be careful of the house plant, which looks similar to Melilot (it's called Colocasia), but it's poisonous.*** Use herbs only from certified and trusted sources!

Preparation: the daily dosage of this tea is prepared with 2 Tbsps. Melilot soaked for 2-3 hours in 2 cups hot water. Strain the infusion, divide it into 2-3 equal parts and take before a meal.

Senna (Senna alexandrina) – the classical anti-constipation herbal remedy. I will mention this herb briefly – it deserves our attention when talking about bowel movement. This plant contains lots of compounds beneficial for us - anthraquinone glycosides called sennosides (and their active substances - chrizofanol, gum anthraquinones, and flavones); tartaric acid salts; bitter substances; resin, and around 10% mucilage. This is one of the strongest laxatives known to men, so be careful with it. The infusion will stimulate the walls of the colon and cause contractions, which evacuate the feces and even some colon parasites. Do not make the tea too strong for it may cause colic pains and cramps. Start with small quantities to test the reaction – the first laxative signs may occur after several hours of consumption. This plant is not suitable for regular use – drink Senna tea not longer than 10 consecutive days for extreme cases of constipation, or consult with your physician. It is little known fact, that Senna is a popular plant in Ayurvedic natural medicine. The plant is used for skin inflammations, some eye conditions, jaundice, liver conditions, bronchitis, anemia, typhoid fever, etc.

Preparation: soak 1 tsp. of the herb in 250 ml (1 cup) hot water for 5 minutes. Strain the infusion and the Senna laxative tea is ready.

Precautions when using Senna tea: this plant should not be taken by young children (especially under 2 years old), and pregnant women. Do not overdose and do not take for longer than 10 days. Senna is also not suitable for severe issues of the

digestive tract and the intestines - ulcers, colitis, diverticulitis, bowel obstructions, inflamed colon and/or appendix. In cases of sensitivity to the active substances in the herb or when overdosing, the side effects can be serious – nausea, stomach cramps, mucus diarrhea, flatulence, dehydration, hypotension, etc. As a recap – be really careful when taking Senna, and use as a last resort for stimulating the bowel movement.

FINAL WORDS

"Prevention is better than cure"
~Desiderius Erasmus Roterodamus

Strengthening the immune system in a natural way is extremely important for our overall health, well-being, and vitality. Wouldn't it be wonderful, if we could evade all diseases? To live a fulfilling, active, and vibrant life, instead of dreading the days of the usual winter flu?

Yes, we all want that, because without health all our dreams and goals become much harder, if not impossible! But our society has been taught to wait for the disease to come and then – "just take this little pill and you will be fine".

In comparison, the ancient wisdom of the Eastern natural medicine concentrates largely on the prevention. It is easier to sustain the good shape of our bodies, to help them cope with the environment on their own, rather than trying to repair the damage. Because sometimes the damage can be irreparable. But as you may already know, I am not here to scare you. On the contrary, my ultimate goal is to give you options and solutions – a natural and safe way out of a problem. And one of the best things we can do for ourselves, for our health, and for our family, is to concentrate on building our innate defense mechanism. I know it is not a 3-day wonder – it requires time, effort, persistence, and consistency. Start slowly; add small habits to your daily routines – some lemon/honey/ginger mix in the morning, maybe some contrasting showers, a yoga sequence every other day, more fresh fruits and veggies, less toxins, a nice warming soothing cup of tea before bed... The options are countless – just choose the ones that are compatible with your lifestyle and health condition, the ones that resonate with you, and experiment! Taking care of our precious bodies and souls is an ongoing process, so that we have the energy and capacity to go after our dreams, to take care of our families, and to enjoy life to the fullest!

Let the ultimate health be with you!

Thank you!

I want to thank you for purchasing this book and reading it all the way to the end. I hope it has been helpful and informative. If you liked this volume, you can support my work and make it more visible for others who are looking for this kind of knowledge! I would deeply appreciate if you take a minute and write a short review on Amazon. I thank you in advance for your support!
Kind regards and best wishes,
Milica

P.S. And don't forget to get your free ebooks:
"10 Powerful Immune Boosting Recipes"
"12 Healthy Dessert Recipes"
"15 Delicious & Healthy Smoothies"
"The Complete Ayurveda Detox"

Go to ***www.MindBodyAndSpiritWellbeing.com*** and claim your gifts!

Or simply scan the QR code below:

About the author

Milica Vladova dedicated her work to spread the valuable knowledge of the physical, emotional, and spiritual wellbeing. She is determined to make the world healthier, happier, and more successful!

Her work has been published on ***The Huffington Post***, ***The Elephant Journal,*** ***Thrive Global***, ***Steven Aitchison***, ***BuzzFeed***, and more.

She is the author of "***The Detox and Strong Immunity Series***", the "***DIY Homemade Beauty Products Series***", and "**The Healthy Vegan Diet Cookbook**".

Find her on:
http://**MindBodyAndSpiritWellbeing.com**
https://facebook.com/**MindBodySpiritWellbeing**
https://www.pinterest.com/**MilicaVladova**
https://twitter.com/**Holistic_Milky**

Milica is also the author of:

★★★★★ Simple and descriptive

I have been trying to get rid of unnecessary chemicals in my life. This book helps me to do just that.
I was looking for DIY shampoo and conditioner; the ingredients are not hard to find.
I love this book! *Thank you Milica Vladova!*

~ Jhitt on Amazon.com

★★★★★ Excelent book

It's very informative and cover a wide range of products.

~ Marisa on Amazon.com

★★★★★ Powerful, holistic detox programme

This book is a treasure for anyone serious about finding natural alternatives to all the harmful things our bodies crave due to the power and pressure of modern life and unscrupulous advertising techniques. If, like me, you are addicted to the sugar and salt added to any processed foods, this book will help wean you into a more energized, natural lifestyle. This fascinating book provides an easily accessible summary of all the major ailments resulting from a "convenience-store" lifestyle. Ms Vladova explains each harmful element in sufficient detail that even those who have researched the subject will find something new. Her comprehensive suggestions (again with just the right level of easy-to-understand explanation) to replace these toxic substances and habits, gives every reader a wide choice of alternatives to suit their budget, lifestyle and preferences. This is so much more than just another diet fad - Ms. V's holistic approach covers so aspects of daily life and outlines good practices which will have immediate beneficial effects.

Using these techniques, my 8-day detox programme resulted in a weight loss of 11lbs, and 5 inches round my waist. *What is more encouraging is that these losses have been maintained 6 weeks later by adjusting my diet and exercise routine according to her advice.*

~ FireDancer on Amazon.co.uk

★★★★★ This is a wonderful, easy to read book loaded with lots of important, but simple information!! I recommend this book for anyone.

The book held my complete attention. I couldn't put it down. I am sure you will find some ideas that you can start implementing right away.

~ Jan Waters on Amazon.com

The Healthy Vegan Recipes Cookbook

***** MORE THAN 80 HEALTHY VEGAN RECIPES FOR THE WHOLE FAMILY! *****

In this volume you will find:
- *Healthy vegan* ***main course dishes;***
- ***Bread and salty snacks*** *recipes.*
- ***Dips*** *and side dishes.*
- *Yummy* ***sugar-free desserts****.*
- *Interesting info about the* ***numerous benefits of vegan foods****.*
- *and much more!*

"The Healthy Vegan Recipes Cookbook" is your guide to the world of healthy vegan cooking!

Printed in Great Britain
by Amazon

57980296R00122